June 2012

CW00798585

The Complete Guide to Precision Reflexology

To Carol,

Best wishes

Jan

The Complete Guide to Precision Reflexology

Second Edition

by Jan Williamson

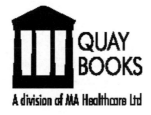

QUAY BOOKS

A division of MA Healthcare Ltd

Quay Books Division, MA Healthcare Ltd, St Jude's Church, Dulwich Road, London
SE24 0PB

British Library Cataloguing-in-Publication Data
A catalogue record is available for this book

© MA Healthcare Limited 2010
ISBN-10: 1 85642 410 3; ISBN-13: 978 1 85642 410 3

Printed by CLE, Huntingdon, Cambridgeshire

Contents

To Ben, John and Patrick

An old Japanese foot tale

Otau was a wise, old and wrinkled man. The whole village respected his healing abilities.
One day a foreigner came to ask him many questions and write down the healing ways of Otau.
However, all Otau would say was, "See to their feet and you have seen to their body"
"I do not understand, " insisted the foreigner.
"Your understanding will never be enough," Otau chuckled. "See to their feet and that will be enough"

Acknowledgements

My deepest thanks to Prue for her trust and great generosity.

Thanks also to Jennifer and Angela for help with the photographs and to John J. Wiliamson for his artwotk. The reflexology charts in this book are produced by kind courtesy of Prue Miskin.

Preface

The aim of this book is to introduce a specific style of reflexology, to explain how and when it can be given and to establish its position within the field of complementary therapies. Hopefully, I will also share my enthusiasm for a therapy that I have found, within clinical practice, to be extremely effective. Perhaps then it is also no coincidence that it is enjoyable both to give and to receive.

Reflexology, along with other therapies, is constantly developing and growing, as is my approach to it. This book represents my perceptions at this time. There are many valid and effective approaches to reflexology, precision reflexology being one of them. This is not a definitive guide but, rather, just one step along the way.

There is, within the world of reflexology, a constant debate about the variety of different charts or "maps" used. To put this into perspective we need to be aware that when reflexology originated 5000 years ago in the East, there was no need for a chart, each treatment being a response between the practitioner's sensitivity and intuition and the recipient's energy levels. This continues to be the underlying principle behind treatments today. The reality of the reflexes is in the practitioner's fingers. The charts are a Western influence, they are necessary as a guide to student learning – but they are simply that, a guide. Given time, students develop and learn to trust their own sensitivity.

Precision reflexology requires therapists to develop their sense of touch, connecting with the client on an energetic level and responding appropriately, aiming to restore a natural equilibrium.

Introduction to the Second Edition

I am delighted that the first edition of "A Guide to Precision Reflexology" has been so enthusiastically received since its initial publication and it has travelled, with the tuition of precision work, around the world to various countries including, Australia, America, the Netherlands, Spain, Denmark, Finland, Belgium and, of course, the U.K. It has now been translated into German and both French and Spanish editions are currently being planned.

Students of both full practitioner training and continuing professional development courses have found the book to be invaluable, especially so because it is the only book available on the subject.

The change in title to "The Complete Guide to Precision Reflexology" reflects the comprehensive coverage of both the basic and new advanced techniques. I am so pleased to be asked to compile this updated version because it gives me the opportunity to share the advanced techniques that I have been developing over recent years. I have been using these in my own practice with clients experiencing positive results and am now teaching them as advanced techniques. I have called this approach "The Unseen Feet" and it offers a way to work with subtle body energy within the framework of massage whilst still using the powerful medium of the feet. More importantly, it involves the client, in practical ways, so that they can become involved in their own holistic health care.

It is a way of working that suits me and I hope you find it interesting.

Jan
February 2010

CHAPTER 1

Reflexology

While the practice of reflexology as a relatively recent development in the field of complementary therapy in the Western world, it is an ancient holistic healing technique derived from oriental philosophy. This philosophy regards the human being as a miniature version of the universe. Man forms an organic part of and is clearly linked to nature. The terminology used by reflexologists such as balance, harmony and energy do not translate easily into Western physiological understanding.

Reflexology is based on the premise that energy channels run throughout the body. The efficacy of the therapy is believed to be the result of stimulation of this energy flow. It is essential to have a basic understanding of this phenomenon. The Indian Yogis call it "prana", the Chinese call it "chi", in the West homeopaths have called it "vital energy" and "life force". Reflexology deals with this internal energy and accepts that the body is a dynamic energy system which is constantly changing.

Oriental belief is that all life is linked to natural rhythms and laws of the universe. The health of each individual depends upon a balance in the natural world, while the health of each organ depends upon its relationship to all other organs. Nothing can change without changing the whole. Humans are directly and indirectly affected by the cosmic forces that are beyond our control. The optimum state is that each individual should live in harmony with nature and the environment. The aim of reflexology, along with other holistic therapies, is to connect to a person's energy system, to adjust it and harmonise it with the world in which that person lives.

All life can be said to be an expression of energy. In human beings this shows itself in various forms – spiritual, emotional, mental and physical. These are all one and the same energy. Holistic therapies acknowledge that imbalances in one level of energy affect other levels and they aim to restore balance within the entire system.

As a holistic healing technique (the term holistic is from the Greek word "holos" which means whole), reflexology treats each individual as an entity of body, mind and spirit. It does not treat symptomatically and does not work on a specific system in a technical manner but, rather, it works with the whole person. The aim being to restore the individual into a state of balance. Because the nature of the whole is always different from the mere sum of its parts, the whole system cannot be properly understood by studying individual parts. It is vital to see each person as an integrated organisation.

Reflexology seems to open up energy channels in the body. Specific techniques are used to apply pressure to the feet which allows energy to circulate throughout the body.

History

Leonardo da Vinci (1452–1519) said that the feet are "a masterpiece of engineering and a work of art" (see *Figure 1.1*). The feet certainly have a special place and a fascination in mythology, religion and culture over the centuries. In mythology the famous reference is that of Achilles' heel, meaning a vulnerable area. The removal of shoes at the threshold of holy places for the Buddhists, the Hindus and the Muslims is compulsory. The North American Indians also regard the feet with high esteem. A Cherokee, Jenny Wallace, a modern day healer and reflexologist in America, says,

"The feet walk upon the earth and through this your spirit is connected to the universe. Our feet are our contact with the earth and the energies that flow through it."

Among reflexologists it is a widely held theory that reflexology originated in China some 5000 years ago, and there is Egyptian documentation dating from around 2500–2300 BC. In the tomb of Ankhmahor, a highly respected physician, there are wall paintings showing what appears to be the practice of reflexology (see *Figure 1.2*). The inscription below the scene reads, "Do not let it be painful" says a patient and the attendant replies "I do as you please". The origins of reflexology are in ancient history when pressure techniques were recognised and accepted as preventative and therapeutic.

The art of reflexology was also known 500 years ago in India. In a Hindu painting of the god Vishnu, the feet symbolise the unity of the entire universe (see *Figure 1.3*). In the same way that Eastern philosophies see the individual being as a microcosm of the universe, so the feet represent the energy of the body.

There is also documentation, dated from the 2nd century BC, describing a Chinese doctor Yu Fu (meaning foot healing) who healed patients with massage.

The earliest records of the European influence on reflexology appear to be in 1582, when Dr Adamus and Dr A'tatis wrote a book on zone therapy. This describes the feet divided into longitudinal zones, with corresponding areas on the body. Western scientific studies in to the neurological function of the body can be traced to Sir Henry Head working in London in the 1890s. He studied the sensory pathways of the body and, with fellow physician, WHR Rivers, he proved the neurological connection between the skin and the internal organs.

At the same time, in Germany, Dr. Alfons Cornelius was working on the fact that pressure points operate within nerve pathways and produce a reaction in a distant part of the body. In 1902 he published a book, "Druckpunkte, or pressure points, their origins and significance".

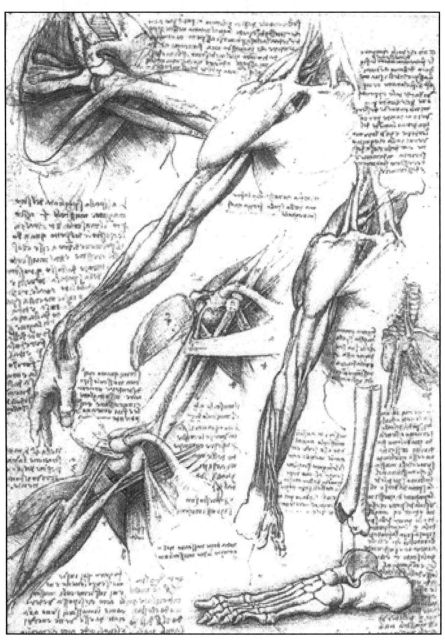

Figure 1.1 Anatomy of arm, shoulder and foot. Circa 1510–11. The Royal Collection ©2010 Her Majesty Queen Elizabeth II .

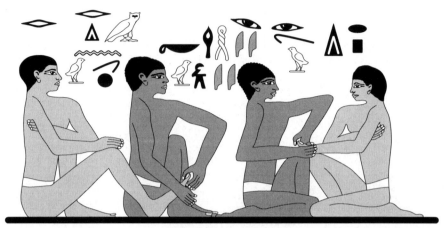

Figure 1.2. Pictograph from tomb of Egyptian physician, Ankhmahor, 2500–2300 BC.

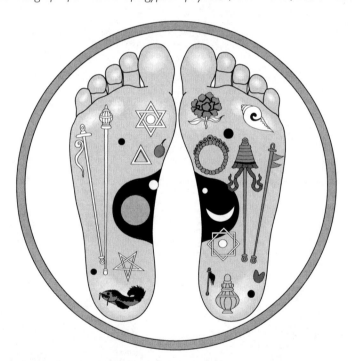

Figure 1.3. Feet of Visnu. India 18th Century.

The American influence came with Dr William Fitzgerald (1872–1942) who "discovered" reflexology while travelling in Vienna at the turn of the century. He was able to show that pressure applied to one area on the foot anaesthetised a corresponding area of the body. This led him to use reflexology in the management of pain. He co-authored a book with a colleague, Dr Edwin Bowers, in 1917 entitled "Zone Therapy". This work was further developed by Dr Joe Shelby Riley who devised a "hooking technique" to apply specific pressure to the feet. He made the first detailed diagrams of the reflex areas located on the feet. A therapist, Eunice Ingham, worked with Dr Riley in America in the 1930s. She made a significant contribution to reflexology with detailed "maps" of the reflex areas of the feet and she wrote two books "Stories the feet can tell" and "Stories the feet have told". In these she explains that, because feet are so responsive to touch, it is possible that, by applying pressure to the various reflexology points on the feet, a definite therapeutic effect can be produced which is far beyond mere pain control.

Sir Charles Sherrington (1861–1952) conducted experiments with the reflex action and coined the term proprioception – meaning how the body's nervous and muscular systems are co-ordinated together. He proved that the entire nervous system responds to external stimulus. At its most reduced level reflexology could be described as an "external stimulus". In 1932, Sherrington was awarded the Nobel prize for his work.

Doreen Bayly, a student of Eunice Ingham, introduced reflexology into Britain in the 1960s. Since then it has become increasingly popular and it is now recognised as a valid form of complementary care.

Rationale

Reflexologists believe that the feet represent the energy of the body. For example, it is believed that the big toe corresponds to the head (see *Figure 1.4*).

The reflex area for the spine is located on the medial aspect of each foot. The reflex areas for the organs and structures of the right side of the body are on the right foot and those of the left side are on the left foot (see *Figure 1.5*).

Reflex areas are on both dorsal and plantar aspects of the feet. The same principles apply to the hands (see *Figure 1.6*).

There are many rationales put forward for reflexology. They reflect its history through Eastern and Western societies. They may refer to the Western influence regarding the neurological and circulatory systems, for example, Doreen Bayly (1978) believed that there is an electrical type impulse triggered by pressure massage on a tender reflex point that can produce a subtle flow of energy, bringing a return to vitality to each person during treatment. Also, Eunice Ingham (1884) said that the nerves of the body can be likened to an electrical system and that reflexology releases tension in that system.

The Eastern approach revolves around concepts of subtle energy,

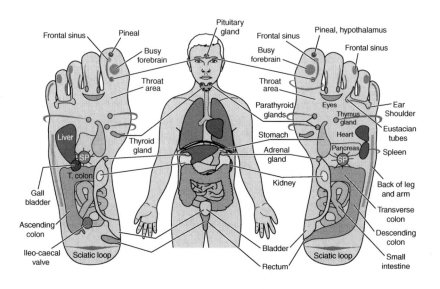

Figure 1.4. Reflexology chart and the relationship to the body.

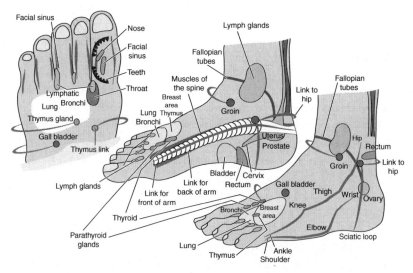

Figure 1.5. Reflex points on the feet.

with reference to chakras and meridians. The aim is to restore the natural equilibrium that the body strives to attain.

We also cannot underestimate the value of receiving undivided attention and care and of promoting deep relaxation, thus providing an optimum situation for the restoration of health.

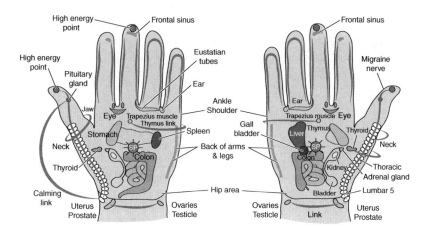

Figure 1.6. Reflex points on the hands.

Application

The reflexology charts are necessary to provide guidance and structure, but rather than being used to deal with one particular symptom, reflexology is used to balance the body's natural equilibrium so that restoration and repair can take place. The Eastern therapeutic approach is that any disease is a result of imbalance, so this therapy is one way to restore that balance and strengthen internal energy.

A thorough knowledge of the location of the reflex areas, of the anatomy and physiology of the body and of the holistic approach to health is required. Practitioners are trained to respond to each treatment with a variety of specific thumb and finger techniques, and to develop sensitivity, so that each consultation is conducted in a caring and responsible manner.

Reflexology can have a positive effect in its ability to relieve stress and tension, whether it be physical or emotional. This often produces an improvement in quality of life. The process of reflexology is not comparable with (diagnostic) methods used in allopathic medicine. Rather, reflexology can be seen as a form of examination which can contribute to an understanding of a condition.

The treatment

As pressure is applied to different reflex points on the feet, different sensations will be felt. A patient's reactions can range from a sharp sensation, to a dull feeling or to a pleasant awareness of pressure. Each treatment is a response to each individual at that time; therefore reactions differ from one person to another and from one treatment to another. One person might experience deep relaxation and another may feel energised. Reflexology is one way, among many, of giving people time to reflect, to relax, to understand their condition and to find some meaning behind it. Rather than suppressing the symptoms, the ethos is to work with the body, both emotionally and physically and to progress accordingly.

Research

There is very little recorded research in reflexology. In 1990, a randomised control trial performed by Lafuente et al (1990) used reflexology in the treatment of headaches. It was a small study, with thirty-two patients randomised to receive drug treatment or reflexology. The study lasted for three months and the results showed that improvements were greater in the reflexology group than in the drug group.

In another study in 1992, Petersen et al examined reflexology in the treatment of asthma. Thirty patients with bronchial asthma were subdivided at random into two groups. One group received ten weekly reflexology treatments and the other had uniform clinical care. A decrease in consumption of medication and an increase in peak flow levels were observed in the group that received reflexology.

In 1994, Oleson and Flocco used reflexology in the treatment of premenstrual symptoms (PMS). This study produced positive results, with a 45% decrease in PMS for the reflexology group and a 20% decrease in a placebo group. In 2002 a study conducted by Exeter University was published which focused on reflexology and menopausal symptoms (Williamson 2002). Both the control group and the placebo group recorded positive results but the difference between the two groups was not scientifically significant and further studies are necessary.

Anecdotal evidence is now no longer sufficient; all complementary therapies deserve high quality research studies. It is possible to conduct this level of study and still remain true to the principles behind complementary care. In this way, solid evidence can be presented to all healthcare professionals. More importantly, it will enable clients/patients to make informed choices about their own healthcare management.

Reflexology had ancient foundations and has evolved into the modern world. It has a rationale which is Eastern in philosophy and Western in application. It has become increasingly chosen as a way of improving and maintaining health in a natural way. Although a popular therapy, it is not claimed to be a magical panacea for all ills but most recipients are able to report some degree of improvement in that it helps to alleviate symptoms or reduces their severity. Patients commonly express feelings of improved well-being. The majority of patients find that treatment reduces stress-related disorders, thus helping them to cope better with the pressures of everyday life.

References

Bayly DE (1978) *Reflexology Today*. Thorsons, Wellingborough: 13–14

Centralised Information for Complementary Medicine. RCCM (research Council for Complementary Medicine), Great Ormond Street, London

Cornelius A (1902) *Druckpunkte*. Berlin

Dougans I, Ellis S (1992) *The Art of Reflexology*. Element Books, Shaftesbury: 10

Fitzgerald Dr. W, Bowers E (1917) Zone Therapy .Mokelumne Hill, CA

Gillanders A (1987) *The Ancient Answer to Modern Ailments*. Ann Gillanders, Harlow: 25–8

Ingham E (1984) *Stories the Feet Have Told*. Ingham Publishing Inc, Saint Petersburg, Florida: 2

Issel C (1990) *Reflexology, Art, Science and History*. New Frontier Sacramento, California: 172

Lafuente A, Noguera M, Puy C, Molins A, Titus F, Sanz F. (1990). *Effekt der Reflexzonendehandlung am Fuss besuglich der priphylattishen Behandlung mit Flunarizin bei an Cephalea-Kopfschmerzen leidenden Patienten. Erfahrungsheilkunde* 1990; 11:713-715

Oleson T, Flocco W (1994) Randomised controlled study of premenstrual symptoms treated with ear, hand and foot reflexology. *Obs Gynaecol* **82**(6): 906–11

Petersen LN, Faurschou P, Olsen OT, Svendsen UG (1992). *Foot zone therapy and bronchial asthma – a controlled clinical trial.* Ugeskr Laeger **154**: 2065-2068

Williamson J et al (2002) Randomised control trial of reflexology for menopausal symptoms. *Br J Obstet Gynaecol* **109**: 1050–5

Precision reflexology

Precision reflexology is one form of reflexology and, as such, it holds the same rationale as other forms of the therapy. It focuses on stimulating "reflex points" on the feet in order to maintain good health. Practitioners believe that, by applying appropriate pressure to these points, it is possible to treat a wide range of disorders. Precision reflexology has been developed by Prue Miskin (founder of the School of Precision Reflexology) during the 1980s and early 1990s. There is a full practitioner training course based on the charts, ethos and style involved with the precision technique. But also, the primary technique, i.e. "linking", can be adapted to other forms of reflexology and it is now extensively taught as a professional development course to practitioners who have trained in other schools.

In order to understand the fundamental principle behind this therapy, it is essential to have an understanding of the origins of all reflexology and, also, of the subtle energy of the body, as explained in Chapter 1. The aim of precision reflexology is to connect to a person's energy system, to adjust it and to harmonise it within itself and with the world surrounding that person. Practitioners work with this internal energy and accept that the body is a dynamic energy system that is constantly changing.

Precision work helps the practitioner to understand the client on all levels. It attempts to make sense of the internal "dialogue" existing within each person. The body has its own multi-directional network of communication. This is not a mechanical process but functions with information and intelligence: it is a form of communication without words.

One important aspect of the unique nature of this technique is that it does not rely on force or actual physical pressure but, rather, it is presented with an element of choice. Each individual client can receive the benefits in a way that is appropriate to him/her at that time. Each person's own energies are used to heal him/herself. It will be appropriate on all levels of clients' being – physical, mental, emotional and spiritual – all these being one and the same energy. Bearing this approach in mind, it is obvious that practitioners must be clear about their own intentions within the treatment; that they are not imposing their will on the client but simply presenting the opportunity for the body to heal itself, using its own innate intelligence. As with all energy work, clearly defined boundaries are important for the safety of both parties. There is a strong, definite connection with "linking" and therapists must ensure that they do not give of their own energy nor take any of the client's energy either. The healing intervention must be allowed to happen in its own way and in its own time. The process of change is not a conscious decision.

An overall guideline throughout is that of acknowledging a condition or presenting symptom and not opposing or denying it. "Success" within the treatment situation is often difficult to define. It may not necessarily mean a lessening or elimination of the original symptom, rather, it can be shown by less obvious, but perhaps more valuable signs, with clients feeling that the quality of their life has improved, or maybe feeling more in control of various aspects of that life. Sometimes a positive outcome can be when recipients of the treatment accept the symptom as a part of themselves and "use" it, asking questions such as, "How does this make me feel?", "Why this particular thing at this time?" or "What does this mean to me?". This approach is obviously quite different from that of Western medicine.

There is a richness to a positive treatment that is difficult to explain; there is no one single formula, each session being a unique response. There are several necessary elements that could be considered:

1. The skill of the practitioner involving technical knowledge and the ability to respond appropriately to reactions felt during the treatment.
2. The energetic overall state of health of the client; the level of harmony within him/herself and with the environment.
3. The unique, complex relationship between the client and the practitioner. Clients need to feel secure, respected, cared for and attended to. Ideally, there is an atmosphere of mutual respect and trust. The aim is to create an optimum environment for recipients to fully engage in the session so that they can begin to feel empowered and to take responsibility for their own health. This daunting task should be a gradual process, allowing time for clients to make appropriate changes to their health care.
4. The experience of the actual treatment can be enjoyable.

Each of these elements reflects the dynamic nature of a treatment, each one responding to another.

Precision reflexology techniques

There are precision reflexology charts that are used in the training of this technique (see Chapter 1). The reflex area for the spine is located on the medial aspect of each foot. Reflex areas are on both dorsal and plantar aspects of both feet. The same principles apply to the hands.

The specific technique which is exclusive to this training is called "linking". This involves holding two (sometimes more) identified reflex points at the same time to add power and definition to the treatment. As the link is held, the therapist pauses and is aware of "listening" via his/her hands and, in this way, the treatment is matched to the individual with precision work. This technique can be adapted to all forms of reflexology and it is currently taught to many students who have qualified in other schools.

"Linking" is initiated by stimulating the reflexes to be connected and feeling the energy between them. Once experienced, this feeling will amplify, especially if both the practitioner and the client are focused. This can be demonstrated on the hands. Points on the thumb and middle finger of each hand are joined together; these are located in the centre of the finger, about a quarter of an inch down from the tip. This vibration can be felt as a tingle, a pulse, a strong beat or a feeling of warmth. There are defined sets of links on the feet and the hands, each producing particular effects and with their own applications; more can also be developed with intuition. Not all of them are for everyone and, in fact, it would not be appropriate to use all the links within a single consultation. The main benefit is that it provides access to the subtle body energies of each client, giving an added dimension to each session and allowing the practitioner to respond fully to the needs of each person.

The treatment is a response to the recipient at that particular time, therefore reactions differ from one person to another and from one treatment to another. The effects produced range from energising and uplifting to calming and deeply relaxing, so the "links" can be used to "match" the needs of the receiver. The treatment reflects the energy levels of the receiver, with some people being more receptive than others. It is possible to balance body energy and the make the therapy truly holistic, both to give and to receive. Experienced therapists can use this approach with accuracy and sensitivity. Awareness of the subtle body increases knowledge of all aspects of a person; physical, emotional and spiritual. In this way, precision reflexology remains true to the Eastern origins of the therapy.

As with all work of this nature, practitioners need to pay attention to their own energy levels and to care for themselves with diet, exercise, relaxation and breathing techniques.

The nature of precision reflexology is that it works with the subtle energy of the body and, as such, it does not respond to strong physical pressure. Each "link" is held with a light touch so a connection can be felt with clear definition but with no force at all. Precision work has the potential for great power even with this gentle pressure and it is particularly effective on painful reflexes or for very fragile and vulnerable clients. The treatment is given without force and it is always presented with great respect for the client. Each person will receive, and progress through, the course of treatment in a way that is correct for them. When, or indeed if, they begin to benefit it will be at the right time for them. This technique then becomes a truly holistic therapy.

There are specific sets of links that will be explained in detail in the following chapters. Here are some general points to bear in mind which apply to all of them:

Reflexology has ancient foundations and has evolved into the modern world. Precision reflexology enables practitioners to remain true to the origins, both in the philosophy behind the treatment and in the approach.

Guidelines to applying links

• The links need to be held while the practitioner "listens" responding to the energy needs of the client. The time to hold will be determined by the needs at that time. After the required time, the worker, and sometimes the receiver too, will feel the response diminish. In this way, the technique is self-regulating; the body taking what it requires.

• The lightest pressure possible is always used while holding the links.

• Sometimes, while holding the link, the practitioner can feel the vibrations that are felt on both reflex points change and occasionally they become equally balanced. At other times, it appears that the energetic contact is therapeutic in itself and the client reports positive reactions following treatment.

• An extremely energetic link on a person who appears to be quite lethargic at the time could indicate an imbalance. However, on a lively, enthusiastic person the same response would be regarded as normal. In the same way, a calm vibration on a link when a person is anxious could be seen as an imbalance while, on a placid, quiet person this would be quite appropriate.

• Each link has its own characteristics, producing its own responses. Clients have a variety of words to describe how they feel, such as "relaxed", "warm", "floaty", "lively", "detached", "energised", and many more. Some of the links can promote feelings of being expansive and free, others of being deeply relaxed. Some can promote emotional release if the client is ready at that time. The technique is received differently by each person, some feeling the responses isolated in the feet, others feeling reactions in the relevant areas of the body. Practitioners make no judgement about this; it is simply how that person is functioning at the time. If a response is felt in the body, clients use words such as "glow", "heat" and "tingle" to describe how this feels.

• Linking can promote deep relaxation, with clients feeling detached from themselves in a physical sense. It emphasises all the benefits of reflexology and can be applied to a wide range of ailments, some physical and others emotional. All complementary health practitioners are aware of how emotional tension after a shock, trauma or bereavement, for instance, can appear to be locked in the physical body as various symptoms present themselves. There are specific links which can, at the right time, help to release this pain. Sometimes this is dramatic with a strong emotional response, sometimes it is calm as the client relates a particular incident from their past.

• There is a stillness to a precision treatment as the links are held. This creates a calm, meditative atmosphere that is beneficial for both client and therapist.

References

Pert CB (1998) *Molecules of Emotion*. Simon and Schuster, USA

Cormack M, Mitchell A (1998) *The Therapeutic Relationship in Complementary Health Care*. Churchill Livingstone, Edinburgh

Mitchell S (1998) *Naturopathy*. Element Books, Shaftesbury

CHAPTER 3

Balance and harmony

Precision reflexology provides a focus for energy work. The Hindu Chakra system (centres of energy) is one way of explaining this concept (see *Figure 3.1*). Chakras do not exist in a physical sense but they give us a way of defining a difficult concept. In a similar way, the Western method of describing a block of energy is to talk about having "a lump in the throat" or "butterflies in the stomach". Each Chakra has many characteristics, including physical, emotional and spiritual qualities; these qualities are all one and the same energy which cannot be separated. This energy can be seen

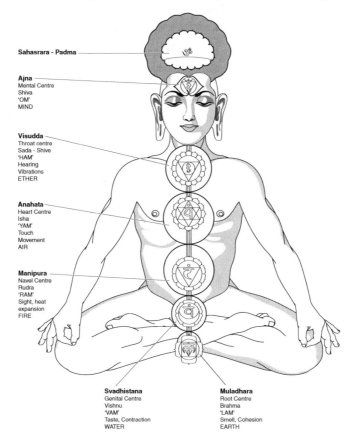

Sahasrara - Padma

Ajna
Mental Centre
Shiva
'OM'
MIND

Visudda
Throat centre
Sada - Shive
'HAM'
Hearing
Vibrations
ETHER

Anahata
Heart Centre
Isha
'YAM'
Touch
Movement
AIR

Manipura
Navel Centre
Rudra
'RAM'
Sight, heat
expansion
FIRE

Svadhistana
Genital Centre
Vishnu
'VAM'
Taste, Contraction
WATER

Muladhara
Root Centre
Brahma
'LAM'
Smell, Cohesion
EARTH

Figure 3.1 The Chakra centres of the body.

as a way of representing the individual within each of us; they are the things that make each of us unique. The relevance to the "linking" technique, and to the endocrine system in particular, is that each Chakra can be said to have a physical counterpart with each endocrine gland. This reinforces the belief that the body registers and feels emotions. Each gland is not only physical but also it holds emotions. Modern Western scientific research has begun to find its own explanations for this phenomenon and Candace Pert (1998) in her book "Molecules of Emotions" says,

"......the key concept is that the emotions exist in the body as informational chemicals, the neuropeptides and receptors, and they also exist in another realm, the one that we experience as feeling, inspiration, love – beyond the physical. The emotions move back and forth, flowing freely between both places and, in that sense, they connect the physical and non-physical. Perhaps this is the same thing that Eastern healers call the subtle energy, or prana – the circulation of emotional and spiritual information throughout the bodymind...My work has taught me that there is a physical reality to the emotions."

The endocrine "links" of precision work can be held, with any imbalances being felt. It would be too prescriptive, too analytical, to focus on one specific link; the ideal approach is to work intuitively with the whole system, aiming for an even distribution of energy throughout. The body's own innate intelligence can be trusted and respected. Each energy centre does not exist in isolation; the entire system is interwoven and is constantly changing, reflecting its dynamics.

However, for reasons of clarity, in this chapter each gland is described in turn, although this is quite artificial as, with the body's remarkable ability, each one is constantly adjusting and responding to activity within its fellow glands. "Linking" attempts, albeit it humbly, to support this connection. The non-physical presentation of this system can provide deeper understanding of an individual and a sense of direction emotionally within a treatment.

Table 3.1 Chakra chart

Chakra	Physical aspect	Non-physical aspect
Sahasrara (Crown)	Pineal gland	Spiritual awareness
Ajna (Brow)	Pituitary gland	Intuition
Vishuddi (Throat)	Thyroid gland	Communication
Anahata (Heart)	Thymus gland	Relationships
Manipura (Solar Plexus)	Pancreas	Confidence
Svadisthana	Adrenal glands	Courage
Muladhara	Gonads	Vitality, security

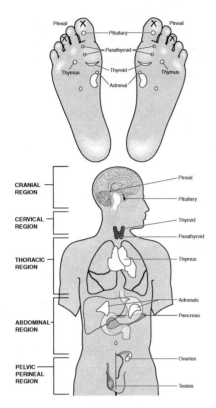

Figure 3.2: The endocrine system of the body and the reflex points on the feet.

Chakra charts

The links associated with the endocrine system are:
1. Thyroid gland to itself
2. Parathyroid glands to themselves
3. Pituitary gland to the adrenal gland
4. Pineal gland to the base of the spine
5. Pituitary gland to the adrenal and the thyroid glands (a 3-way link).

The linking technique reinforces the natural communication processes of this system. *Figure 3.2* shows the reflexes for the endocrine glands.

The thyroid link is located by holding, very lightly, the central point of the thyroid reflex on the plantar aspect with the thumb of one hand and the middle finger of the other hand holding a point, again very lightly, immediately above on the dorsal aspect (see *Figure 3.3*). The dorsal point is held still while the remainder of the plantar thyroid reflex is worked across to the medial line and then back again.

The practitioner can feel a strong pulsating or tingling sensation or, at the other end of the spectrum, a flat or dull response. The client can have a pulsing, rod-like feeling between the two points, and it can feel tender – in which case the pressure needs to be reduced even more. Light touch of a link is more effective than deep pressure. This link can be equally effective for an under-active, or over-active thyroid state because it aims to restore balance. It can be helpful for clients with low energy levels or with any imbalances within the metabolic process. It assists the natural function of the thyroid – and parathyroid – gland, adjusting the levels of calcium in the blood and the bones. Therefore, in cases where the level of this vital mineral is compromised, for example with arthritis and osteoporosis, it can be given special attention.

The parathyroid link is found by holding each plantar reflex in turn and linking each one to itself by holding a dorsal point immediately above (see *Figure 3.4*). This can often feel hot for both the practitioner and the client, with the now familiar possibility of a connection being felt through the foot,

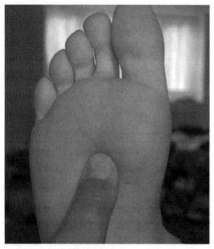

Figure 3.3: The thyroid link.

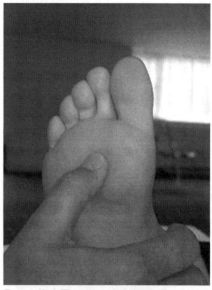

Figure 3.4: The parathyroid link.

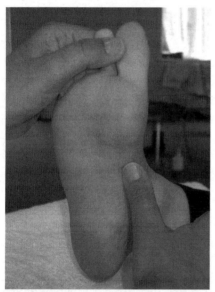

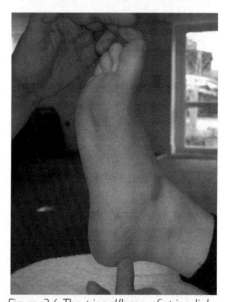

Figure 3.5: The pituitary/adrenal link.   Figure 3.6: The pineal/base of spine link.

this one feeling as fine as a needle. It has an invaluable application, along with the thyroid gland link, because of its ability to assist with the adjustment of calcium levels.

The pituitary gland is "linked" to the adrenal by holding the pituitary with the thumb of one hand and the adrenal reflex with the other thumb (see *Figure 3.5*). Often heat is felt on the adrenal reflex, with a feeling of connection between these two points. This appears to reinforce the natural communication between these two glands, and between the endocrine and nervous systems (because of the adrenal response to stressful situations). This technique can restore balance, having a beneficial effect on the nervous system and creating a feeling of deep relaxation. It has a specific application for menopausal women, assisting with hormonal balance and reducing the over activity of the adrenal glands that sometimes accompanies the menopause; this can help to reduce the severity and frequency of hot flushes and night sweats. Adrenal energy can become depleted as a result of stress, hormonal imbalances or by the consumption of stimulants such as coffee or alcohol, and this energy can be revitalised by this link.

The pineal gland can be "linked" to the base of the spine, simply by holding the pineal reflex with one thumb and the sacrum reflex with the middle finger of the other hand (see *Figure 3.6*). The practitioner can feel this as a circuit of energy or as a sensation of lightening, of releasing. The client often says that this feels "light, as though floaty" and relaxing. It is especially useful at the end of a treatment, as it both seals and closes down the session.

It is possible to apply three-way links, one of these being between the pituitary, adrenal and thyroid glands. It is located by holding the pituitary and adrenal gland reflexes as previously described and then taking the middle finger of one hand to hold the dorsal thyroid reflex (see *Figure 3.7*). This can feel very powerful, with both therapist and client feeling the strong triangle-link connection between the three points. There can be a feeling of heat, or sometimes a sensation of energy "bouncing" from one point to another. It can establish a holding, secure feeling. It is often helpful when clients feel the need to release pent-up emotions. These anxieties may be recent or they may be long-standing, perhaps from childhood. Often the action of verbalising and releasing these concerns is therapeutic in itself. This release will only happen when the individual is ready to do so but, if the practitioner can sense that this is the case, it can mimic the effect of giving someone a hug and allowing him/her to feel secure and safe within the emotional state. It is powerful, encompassing a major portion of a crucial system of the body.

All systems within the body are continually communicating and responding to each other, but the endocrine and nervous systems together have a unique role with the task of maintaining homeostasis, that state of balance that the body strives to be in.

Taking into account the tremendous amount of both internal and external stresses in the modern world, this two-way relationship between hormones and tension levels is amazingly resilient, robust and effective. There is a constant feedback operating within the endocrine system, trying to maintain order. It is an all-powerful structure having an effect on the entire body.

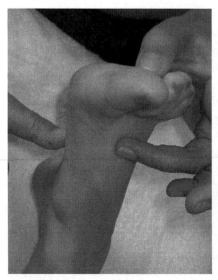

Figure 3.7: The pituitary/adrenal/ thyroid link.

The endocrine system can be seen as the way in which we cope with our environment. It can reflect the level of harmony, within the self, and with the world. When there is an imbalance within this system it is often reported as a feeling of "loss of control" or "not coping". It can feel like an all-encompassing process over which the individual has no control, and an imbalance can produce behaviour and feelings that are quite out of character. This can be, at best, confusing and, at worst, terrifying. Reflexology, at these times, can offer specific help with restoring balance and reducing stress levels. Perhaps, more importantly, the practitioner can also offer reassurance and support and give realistic self-help advice so that individuals can begin to feel in control of themselves again.

Case studies

1. Client details – Hazel. Age 52. Married. One grown-up daughter. Runs local shop.

Presenting symptom: Menopausal hot flushes. She feels that these dominate her life; she has several overnight, resulting in very disturbed sleep for herself and her husband. She also has frequent hot flushes during the day, sometimes so severe that she has to leave the room and go outdoors. These now restrict her social life. She is determined not to take hormone replacement therapy (HRT), wanting to manage the menopause naturally.

Treatment: On presentation all the endocrine and reproductive reflexes felt hot and tender. The neck area was tight with the neck to jaw link (see Chapter 4) feeling very energetic to the practitioner, so this was held several times during the treatment. The pituitary to adrenal link was also worked, with heat felt on the adrenal. There was a steady improvement for the first four weekly sessions, with the heat on the adrenal reflex gradually reducing and, at the same time, Hazel felt that the night-time sweats were less severe. After the fourth session, the symptoms worsened for a short time but, after the sixth treatment there continued to be a steady improvement. At this time, the hot flushes reduced both in severity and frequency. The usual pattern then was just one which she was aware of overnight but not enough to disturb sleep, and perhaps two or three during the day but, as she said, "They are manageable". She felt delighted and confident to allow the menopause to progress naturally and continued to have regular monthly treatment to sustain the improvement. She continued to thoroughly enjoy the sessions and said, "It does work but, even if it didn't, I would still come because it feels wonderful."

Incidentally she realised after several sessions that she had not needed to make the regular appointment with the osteopath because she had had no neck problems.

2. Client details – Joyce. Age 35. Married with three young children.

Presenting symptom: Premenstrual syndrome. This lasts for two weeks before each period when she feels irritable and depressed. This feels alien to her because she normally has a positive attitude to life. She feels tired all the time.

Treatment: She was intrigued and fascinated by the full treatment she received which gave particular focus to the entire endocrine system. The thyroid reflex point felt dull and very flat on the left foot. The pituitary to adrenal, thyroid and parathyroid links were all worked. The small intestines reflex was also tender and tight.

She received four weekly treatments, then the interval was extended to fortnightly for four more sessions, and then regular monthly sessions were established. After the sixth treatment, she felt an improvement in her overall energy levels and after three months she felt that there had been a gradual reduction in the severity of the pre-mentrual syndrome (PMS). This is now an occasional problem, not associated with every period and only lasting for three or four days. She values the consultation time as her only relaxation in a very busy schedule.

3. Client details – Josephine. Age 36. Single. Lives alone except for her small dog. No children. She is unemployed, having had to retire for health reasons.

Presenting symptoms: Myalgic encephalomyelitis (ME) for five years. She has disturbed sleep patterns, only being able to sleep for two or three hours at a time. She tends to sleep both throughout the day and night and she has no social life. Her concentration levels are low and she feels that she has no energy at all. She experiences muscular pain and feels frustrated and uncoordinated because she wants to move but finds it hard, sometimes impossible, to do so.

Treatment: At the first treatment, the practitioner felt strong reactions with some of the links, namely the neck to jaw and lumbar 5 to hip (see Chapter 4). These were worked several times during the treatment although each time the client felt very little. She did feel that the pituitary reflex was tender so this was worked gently. The pressure throughout was very light and Josephine relaxed and feel asleep after thirty minutes. At the second treatment, one week later, Josephine reported feeling exceptionally tired after the initial treatment and had, in fact, slept for almost twenty four hours. She needed reassurance that, hopefully, this would not happen after every session. Attention was given to the pituitary/adrenal link with a view to boosting energy; this felt quite vibrant to touch and the client felt a connection between the two reflexes which she described as a "red, dotted line". Again a strong reaction was felt by the practitioner on the neck/jaw and lumber 5/hip links. Josephine relaxed and slept again. One week later, at the third session, she felt more positive in general and looked brighter. For two nights in the week she had slept for a longer period of time and was, therefore, awake for longer in the daytime. The pineal to base link was held with a view to adjusting melatonin levels. When the lumber 5/hip link was held, Josephine felt a connection between the two points and also a tingling sensation moving up her leg. She felt encouraged by this saying, "Perhaps there is some life in my legs after all."

The fourth treatment was two weeks later and Josephine looked more alert and was smiling. She was very pleased with herself having managed to walk her dog, instead of having to ask a neighbour and she was sleeping better with clearer distinctions between the day and night time. Again she felt some referred sensations with some of the links.

She continued with monthly treatments for three months and then settled to six-weekly sessions. The ME remains a major part of her life but she usually manages a daily walk and, because of her improved sleep pattern, she can organise a social life, albeit quite limited. In appearance she continues to look brighter and smiles more. She still has periods of depression but feels that these are less severe. From time to time she talks about childhood problems, notably a difficult relationship with her father. She sees the reflexology consultations as a way of "off loading" and helping her to cope. She has started to attend a yoga class and feels the benefits from this, both physical and emotional.

4. Client details – Mabel. Age 67. Married. Busy. Loves organising.

Presenting symptom: Arthritis in both knees.

Treatment: On presentation, the neck and shoulders were very tight and tense. The neck to jaw link (see Chapter 4) was held and she commented that this felt uncomfortable. The thyroid and parathyroid links were also held with a view to increasing bone calcium levels. Mabel found it difficult to relax, she didn't close her eyes at all and talked throughout the session. She was interested in the effect of diet on her condition, this being a new concept for her, and she discussed with the practitioner how she could reduce acid-forming food realistically. At the second session her feet felt more relaxed, although the neck to jaw link was still powerful and tender. She was quiet for a short time. At the third treatment she talked about her grand-daughter and then started to talk about herself as a child, about her brother and also about her strict father who had often made her feel frightened and angry. As she talked, her feet, and then the rest of her, began to relax. The pituitary/adrenal/thyroid link was being held gently and she seemed to soften and smiled more (instead of frowning).

At subsequent treatments, usually at monthly intervals, she relaxed after a short time and closed her eyes. The neck and shoulder reflexes became less tense each time. She commented that it was "wonderful just to be able to talk about myself". She still has some pain in her knees but manages to enjoy her garden with help and her overall appearance is brighter.

Reference

Pert CB (1998) *Molecules of Emotion*. Simon and Schuster, New York: 307

CHAPTER 4

Framework

To attach meaning to the consultations, it is necessary to remember that two of the main functions of the skeleton are:

- Movement
- Protection.

If someone has a problem with the framework of their body they understandably feel vulnerable with a loss of protection and control. This is especially so if it is a spinal problem, with the person feeling that the very core of their being is damaged. Reduced movement produces feelings of frustration and depression and often the associated pain is debilitating in itself. These feelings can be addressed within the actual hands-on treatment; if a client is feeling depressed and low then a stimulating treatment to lift the spirits would be appropriate. The relationship between each person and the practitioner can also help emotionally. The aim is for clients to feel respected and cared for; in this supportive environment they can begin to feel in control of various aspects of their health. The manner and context of the dialogue need not be intense or daunting but, rather, relaxed and conversational in style. Some individuals may welcome an opportunity to discuss emotional problems, for others it may be more appropriate to discuss realistic ways to take charge of their own health in practical ways, eg. dietary changes or a gentle exercise programme. A positive outcome would be for the client to be involved in, and confident with, their own healthcare.

The "links" influencing the skeleton system are:

- Neck to jaw
- Lumbar 5 to hip
- Leg and arm work.

The whole length of the spine is worked (see *Figure 4.1*), using circular movements of the thumb or middle finger to locate the reflex point for each vertebrae. Gentle yet effective pressure

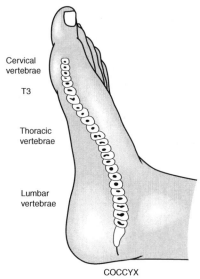

Cervical vertebrae

T3

Thoracic vertebrae

Lumbar vertebrae

COCCYX

Figure 4.1: Spinal reflexes on the feet.

27

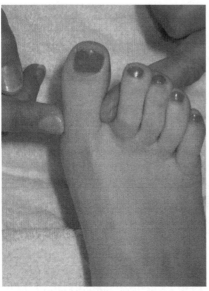

Figure 4.2: The neck to jaw link.

is used with particular attention being given to sensitive areas.

For any neck condition, pain and tension in the jaw or for tension headaches, the neck to jaw link can be used (see *Figure 4.2*). The reflex for cervical 5 is linked to the jaw reflex inside the big toe. This is particularly effective for people who have tension in their jaw, or for those who grind their teeth. It is an easy link to locate, with the practitioner often feeling a pulsating sensation on either or both of the points. Often heat is felt by the practitioner and/or the client. The client often reports feeling a connection through, or around, the big toe. The importance of this link is that, in reflexology, it is frequently painful to work directly on the neck reflex but, with a light touch, this technique is both effective and powerful.

A powerful link is lumbar 5 to the hip reflex (see *Figures 4.3 and 4.4*). The 5th lumbar vertebrae reflex point (on the medial aspect) is held and linked to the hip reflex point (on the lateral aspect). This is particularly effective for any hip or knee conditions or for conditions affecting the sciatic nerve. It has a relaxing effect on the nervous system so that it can be applied to any stress-related problems.

This can be amplified further by transferring it into a three-way link by holding the mid-point of the sciatic loop on the plantar aspect (see *Figure 4.5*). This has a specific application for conditions affecting the sciatic nerve.

The connection between the lumbar spine and the hip represents an area of the body that is full of activity, ie. the pelvis. The link reflects the energetic sense of the client, sometimes with the practitioner feeling a strong, pulsating energy and sometimes a calm, light response. The treatment is presented with no sense of judgement so neither

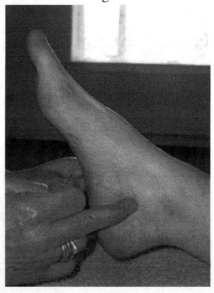

Figure 4.3: The lumbar 5 to hip link.

is right or wrong but it matches the person at that time, with the aim being, as with all reflexology, to find a balance.

In common with some of the other links, the lumbar 5 to hip can generate a feeling of heat and a sense of connection through the foot. The client can report feeling the same rod-like connection, also sometimes a tingling sensation moving up the leg, perhaps to the hip or into the spine. This tends to be directed to where it is needed the most so, for instance, it may be described as warmth moving around the knee or around the hip and then returning back down to the foot. The energy can regulate itself and fade

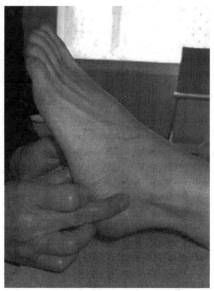

Figure 4.4: the lumbar 5 to hip link.

away when appropriate – with both the client and the practitioner feeling this. Each person's reactions to the links are unique, with some people feeling referred sensations in the body and others feeling very little; neither is correct or incorrect but rather it represents how that person is functioning at that time. As clients relax into this procedure, the words that have been used to describe it include "floating", "lightening" and "opening out" – these appear to be accurate ways of outlining a release of tension with our limited Western vocabulary. Often it can feel very comforting to have the foot held in this way.

Precision reflexology has an interesting procedure for working the reflexes for the legs and arms using the linking technique. For the leg, the lumbar 5 reflex is held while the middle finger of the other hand traces the outline of the leg on the lateral aspect of the foot (see *Figure 4.6*). The outline goes from the hip, down the back of the leg to the ankle and then back up again, over the kneecap, into the groin and back to the hip.

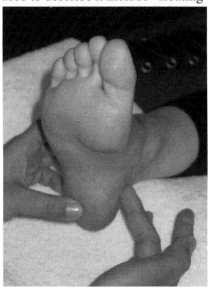

Figure 4.5: The lumbar 5/hip/sciatic loop.

The arm is worked by holding the

point for thoracic 3 on the spinal reflex and linking across to the shoulder reflex on the lateral aspect of the foot. Please note that this link in itself can have very positive results when treating shoulder problems such as "frozen shoulder". Whilst still holding the thoracic 3 point, the outline of the arm goes from the shoulder, down the outside of the arm to the wrist and then back up again, via the elbow to the armpit. The "circuit" is then completed by working across the foot to the jaw and holding the neck/jaw link again (see *Figure 4.7*).

This method for leg and arm work amplifies the effects of treatment.

Within a treatment, the whole length of the spine is worked. Initially, the jaw link is held with the middle finger of one hand, as small circular pressure is applied along the cervical vertebrae with the middle finger of the other hand. Then the jaw point is released and this finger is placed lightly on the top of the big toe and remains there while the other hand works along the length of the spine down to the coccyx. When working the spine each vertebra is located so that the treatment is very focused and detailed. Then the leg and arm work follows as detailed above.

Using linking to work the spine amplifies a treatment, increases sensitivity and often creates dramatic connections within the actual spine. Using small circular strokes, it is possible to detect precisely each individual vertebra. Sensitive areas may reflect structural problems or neurological ones, often indicating an imbalance within an organ which has its nerve intervention at that point. At any tender spots, the reflex is lightly held in order to increase the effectiveness. This can be assisted by guiding the client

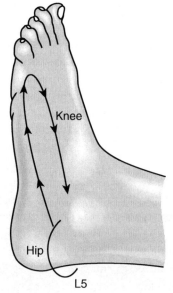

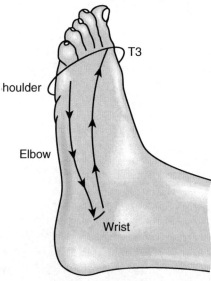

Figure 4.6. Left reflexes on the feet.   *Figure 4.7 Arm reflexes on the feet.*

through appropriate breathing techniques, to direct the breath to a particular area. Using this approach, the experienced practitioner can feel a variety of responses which can mirror how the client is feeling. The information that can be picked up from this spinal work is significant, as it usually matches the nature of the client, with tender areas often reflecting emotion sensitivities.

Case study

Client details – James. Age 61. Retired clerical officer. Married.

Presenting symptom: Arthritis in the knees. When describing how he feels about this, James says that he feels "cheated" because he was looking forward to enjoying an active retirement. He experiences pain and stiffness in the morning and he feels afraid to walk for any distance in case the pain levels increase.

Treatment: He received a full treatment at each session, with the focus on the solar plexus area for pain relief, on the adrenal reflexes in order to try to stimulate the body's natural anti-inflammatory response and also (thinking about the fight/flight reaction) to address the feelings of fear. The primary links would be the lumbar 5 to knee (as part of the procedure for working the leg) and, also, the thyroid and parathyroid links (see Chapter 3).

Initially James found it difficult to relax; he talked a lot during the first treatment and had his eyes open throughout. At the first consultation there was a realistic discussion about his health. He was not looking for, or expecting, a cure but he was reassured by a positive outlook of hopefully slowing down the progress of his condition. Dietary recommendations were also discussed, with the aim of reducing acid-forming foods, ie. concentrated proteins. He talked about realistic ways in which he could achieve this yet still have a diet that he would enjoy. To assist with the removal of toxins, and to improve his overall circulation, he was guided through a basic deep breathing routine. This approach was completely new to him but he felt much brighter and, in his own words, "at least there is something that I can do for myself".

He was intrigued by the feel of the linking technique. The lumbar 5 to knee produced an especially strong response and he described feeling a definite tingle in his knees. This in itself boosted his morale; he said that it reassured him that there was "life in there still".

After four sessions at fortnightly intervals, he reported that the pain had reduced in the mornings. He felt more confident and was taking gentle walks each day. He relaxed during the treatments now. He had started to make plans for his retirement and had started to garden again.

CHAPTER 5

Movement

The muscles of the body provide strength and mobility, so any problems can produce feelings of weakness, frustration, heaviness and, at times, depression. We can move from the day that we are born and, when this ability is compromised, naturally our spirits can be deeply affected. As previously described, these feelings can be addressed in the wider aspects of the consultation – including the benefits of the client/practitioner relationship, the relaxation that is promoted by the treatment and any self-help healthcare that can be generated.

For some conditions it can be very therapeutic, in the acute stage, to realise the benefit of rest with a gradual introduction of gentle exercise. This process alone often allows the person concerned to learn to care for him/herself with awareness.

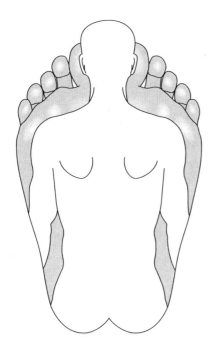

Figure 5.1: Muscular framework of body in relation to reflex points.

Just as the feet represent the energy of the whole body, the entire muscular system has reflex points on the feet (see *Figure 5.1*). In a standard treatment the whole of the foot is worked (as described in Chapter 13) and all the muscles are given attention. The reflexes for the muscles of the spine can be specifically worked by applying circular thumb pressure to either side of the spinal reflex for its full length.

The specific link for this system is :
• Shoulder link – plantar reflex point is linked through to a dorsal point immediately above (see *Figure 5.1*).

A reflex point at the base of the fourth toe on the plantar aspect of the foot is held using one thumb, with the middle finger of the other hand holding a point immediately above on the dorsal aspect. This is effective for muscular problems of the shoulder area. Often

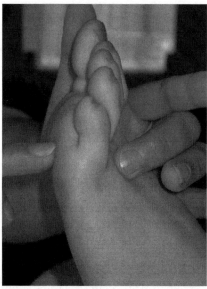

Figure 5.2: Shoulder link.

both the practitioner and the client feel heat with this link and either, or both, may be aware of a rod-like connection through the foot. The client may need reassurance about this feeling and deep breathing exercises practised at the same time can be beneficial.

Emphasising the importance of every aspect of the spine, the muscles here are involved with the overall health of the person. When treating a client who presents with a shoulder or arm condition, the practitioner can often feel tension and restriction in the reflex point for the thoracic muscles. Likewise, with a client who has a pelvic or leg problem, a similar response can be felt in the lumbar reflexes. This is one of the strengths of reflexology, in that it can help to find the root cause of a problem. Often, when working the reflexes for the spinal muscles, a clients' breathing will deepen and they become more relaxed, thus assisting with the overall situation.

Case study

Client details – Norma. Age 47.

Married with two children (one married daughter and one son at university). She cares for her elderly mother who is becoming increasingly dependent. She is a teacher, which she used to enjoy but with which she is now dissatisfied and says, "This is not the job that I trained to do."

Presenting symptoms: Pain in her left shoulder. Headaches, which she herself feels are a result of the shoulder tension.

Treatment: On presentation, both the right and left shoulder reflexes were tight and tender with this being more pronounced on the left side. She obviously received a full treatment with particular attention being given to the solar plexus, neck and small intestines, all of which felt tense and tight. The muscular shoulder link was held through the foot. Gentle pressure was applied and this link was repeated several times during the treatment. The neck to jaw link (see Chapter 4) was also used: the light touch was especially appropriate here because of the tenderness in this area. All the reflexes around the head area were very erratic and a focus within the session was to calm these down. She valued this time for herself and felt that she had been given "permission to be still" for one hour – which she described as "bliss".

After the first treatment the shoulder pain worsened for two days and then eased. This was followed by three further consultations, at weekly intervals, after which time the shoulder pain was consistently reduced and the headaches were less frequent and less severe. She continues to attend at monthly intervals and the relationship between her and the practitioner has developed into one of mutual trust and respect. Her observations have progressed from saying, "It is so wonderful to have nothing to do for one hour" to a realisation of the benefits of relaxation spilling over into her own time. After three months, she made a conscious decision to care for herself, justifying this by saying that she feels so cared for during the treatments that she should continue this in her own time. Consultation dialogue had centred around appropriate nutrition and the importance of not eating when stressed or hurried, so she set aside time to eat lunch. This involved the co-operation of her colleagues who, incidentally, have started to follow her example. She now attends a weekly keep-fit class, both for the exercise and to give her some time for herself.

She has arranged part-time care for her mother and has come to terms with this, having described to the reflexologist her understandable, but groundless, feelings of guilt and inadequacy. She now accepts that she had previously felt overwhelmed with responsibility but this is now much reduced as she has begun to share these feelings with her husband. So, literally, she has lessened some of the burden from her shoulders.

CHAPTER 6

Communication

The nervous system is the body's communication network, sending messages around to its various parts. Not surprisingly, when people are under stress they often describe themselves as "living on their nerves", or "feeling nervy" and they feel out of control and not connected within themselves or with their environment. The treatment provides an opportunity to break the stress pattern, to go into a state of relaxation. Given time, hopefully, the benefits can extend outside the treatment room and the individual can achieve a sense of control in daily life.

A full reflexology treatment has a beneficial effect on the entire nervous system, promoting deep relaxation; bringing obvious benefits to clients who are experiencing any stress-related problems.

The specific links for this system are:
- Forebrain to sacrum
- Solar plexus to itself.

For the forebrain to sacrum link one thumb holds the forebrain area on the big toe, while the middle finger of the other and holds the sacrum (see *Figure 6.1*). In effect, the conscious thinking part of the brain is connected to the base of the spine. It is ideal for people who find it difficult to unwind and to "switch off" their thoughts. It aims to take the person into a parasympathetic nervous state, facilitating relaxation, creating an optimum situation for the body to heal itself and to strive for homeostasis. Often, for clients who chatter nervously, this link has been known to silence them in mid-sentence. Practitioners can sometimes feel an imbalance between these two points and be aware of a sense of release as the forebrain reflex point calms down. Clients describe this link as feeling "floaty and calming", as though "draining away" the tension.

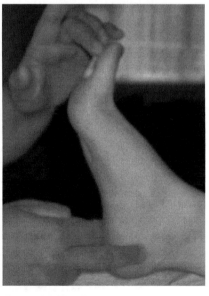

Figure 6.1: The forebrain to sacrum link.

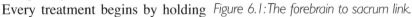

Every treatment begins by holding

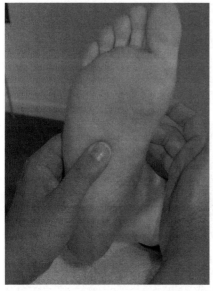

the solar reflex and, in this way, gaining an insight into the nervous state of the person. This link is achieved by holding the plantar solar plexus reflex point with the thumb of one hand and then holding a point directly above, on the dorsal aspect, with the middle finger of the other hand (see *Figure 6.2*). Clients may feel the need for reassurance as they can feel a connection running through the foot between the two points. This link can detect levels of stress, pain and anxiety. For instance, it can feel energetic or dull, delicate or robust, vibrant or calm – all reflecting the recipient in a neurological way.

Figure 6.2: The solar plexus link.

Case study

Client details – Phyllis. Age 42.

Married with two sons aged eleven and thirteen. Her husband works away from home during the week. She is a personel officer who carries a high level of responsibility and stress.

Presenting symptoms: Headaches, which she feels are mainly stress-related, and pre-menstrual syndrome, the worst aspect of which being intense irritability. She also complains of weight gain – she believes this to be hormonal and she has an uncontrollable sugar craving associated with the prementrual syndrome (PMS). She is very organised and controlled with all other areas of her life and feels "ashamed" about this.

She has a bright, extrovert personality, is aware of the stress factors in her life and of how these may be affecting her present state of health.

Treatment: On presentation, the thyroid and neck reflexes were tender, possibly reflecting her tension. The forebrain reflex area felt very erratic and tingly to the practitioner and then become calmer as the link with the sacrum was held. Incidentally, as the course of treatments progressed, the forebrain area became calmer but always powerful – appearing to match the client's life-style.

The first three treatments were at fortnightly intervals and then there were regular monthly sessions. She enjoyed the treatments immediately but did not relax until the third session. After the first two treatments the headaches worsened and then, after the third, they were noticeably reduced, both in severity and frequency. The irritability associated with the PMS has steadily reduced and she now feels that it is manageable.

Within the consultation, she discussed her eating patterns. In order to maintain a steady blood-sugar level, she has organised herself to take time to eat breakfast and a piece of fruit mid-morning (instead of the previous chocolate bar). She now leaves her desk so that she eats in a more relaxed manner at lunch time. This has eliminated the need for a "quick hit" of sugar in the afternoon, and then she has a small evening meal. In addition, also considering the blood-sugar levels, she has gradually reduced her coffee intake. The sugar cravings are far less frequent now. Previously, if she succumbed to the cravings, she felt guilty and, if she resisted them, then she felt resentment. Now, if she eats chocolate she can enjoy it, knowing that it is an occasional treat. As a result, her self-esteem is restored.

She continues with the monthly treatments, feeling the benefit of the "time out" in a very busy life. She reports handling stressful situations in a calmer manner than previously.

CHAPTER 7

Fuel

The functions of the digestive system are ingestion, digestion, absorption, assimilation and elimination of food. It is affected by stress in a very distinctive primitive way. The intestines have a strong relationship with the nervous system and with the emotions – we have all experienced the phenomenon of a "gut reaction" so it could be said that the intestines are themselves emotional when feelings of tension or excitement are evident (see Chapter 16). Unfortunately, modern Westerners generally abuse this system with an over-refined, inadequate diet and often ignore the effect that stress has on the digestive processes. The body is not designed to digest food when in a "fight/flight" situation because other functions of the body are more necessary at that time. The Eastern approach, which says not to eat when you are angry, stressed or hurried is a kinder and more realistic viewpoint.

Eating fresh, whole food is one way of taking charge of one's health. Also, by responding to the information from the digestive process, for example eating only when hungry and resting the system when necessary, demonstrates an awareness of "listening" to the body's messages and of caring for oneself accordingly.

Currently there is much confusion and emotion surrounding food issues. Clients often feel overwhelmed with information and they need reassurance and guidance just to remind them that, primarily, eating ought to be an enjoyable and social event as well as being nutritious.

The reflexes for the digestive system are shown in *Figure 7.1*. The specific link is:
• Gall bladder to itself.

The gall bladder reflex point is held with the thumb of one hand, with the middle finger of the other hand holding a point immediately above on the dorsal aspect of the foot (see *Figure 7.2*).

This can improve the function of the gall bladder, aiding the digestion of fat. It is especially helpful in reducing tension within the entire digestive process.

The stomach reflex is given attention with a circular thumb stroke to cover the whole area. Generally speaking, this organ is quite robust and therefore a firm pressure can be applied – unless the recipient has a stomach disorder, or if it feels tender to touch, then appropriate sensitivity should be used.

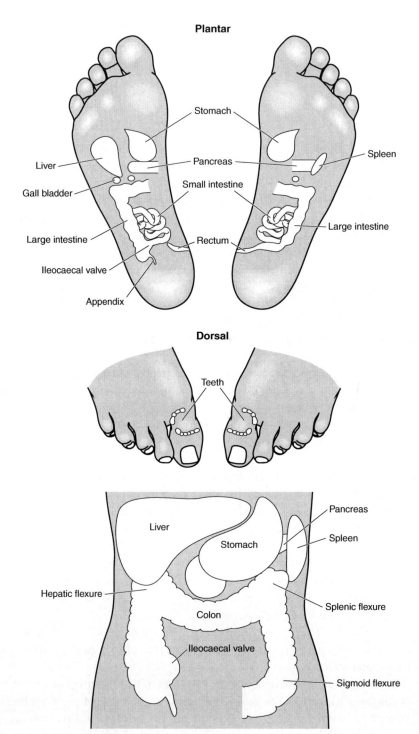

Figure 7.1: Reflexes for the digestive system.

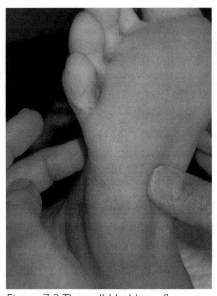

Figure 7.2 The gall bladder reflex.

The same approach applies to the liver reflex, with firm thumb pressure being used to cover the small intestine reflex area unless otherwise indicated. For variety, a different stroke can be used to cover the small intestine area. One stroke that is pleasant to give and to receive is a "fanning" stroke, with both thumbs working horizontally across the foot from side to side, one above the other (see *Figure 7.3*). Also, in order to "scan" the relatively large area of the intestines, a "walking" stroke can be used. This involves moving diagonally over the area with the thumb, the pressure being constant with the joint of the thumb remaining soft as it glides along (see *Figure 7.4*). This can often indicate where more attention is needed and this can then be given with the more specific circular thumb pressure. To cover the large intestine reflex area this same circular thumb stroke is used to move along its length.

As you expect, the nature of the intestinal reflexes often reflects the emotional state of the client, for instance, clients can feel tense and congested or flexible and relaxed.

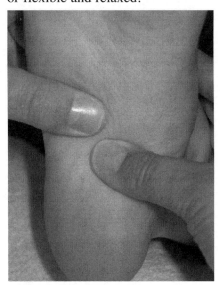

Figure 7.3: Fanning stroke over the small intestine area.

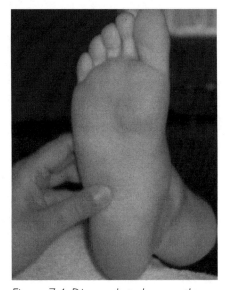

Figure 7.4: Diagonal stroke over the small intestine area.

Case study

Client details – Mavis. Age 32. She is a single parent with two children aged four and two. She is a full-time mother.

Presenting symptom: Irritable bowel syndrome. She experiences abdominal pain and bloating. She has a restricted diet and feels miserable about this. She is slightly overweight.

Treatment: Mavis' initial reaction was one of delight because of having time to herself, to be "pampered" as she said. She received a full treatment so that all the reflexes were worked, with gentle attention to the small and large intestines both of which felt very tight and tender. The gall bladder link was held lightly with the practitioner feeling intense heat. The client relaxed instantly and fell asleep for a short time.

After three treatments, at monthly intervals, she reported that the pain and bloating were both reduced; each time the intestines felt looser and the heat on the gall bladder reflex reduced. At the fourth session she was quite tearful and talked about her feelings of loss and loneliness since her divorce, which she had been unable to express before.

In order to relax and to improve the circulation to the intestines, the reflexologist guided Mavis through deep breathing exercises which she continued to practice daily at home. Also, to improve abdominal tone and to reduce weight, she has included some physical exercise into the daily routine that fit in with family life, either going for a walk or by following an exercise DVD.

She continues with regular monthly treatments. The feet usually show neck and shoulder tension as well as a tight abdominal area but all of these relax during the session. She has also been able to extend her diet and has some completely pain-free spells.

There are occasional lapses which coincide with stressful times but these respond positively to the treatment.

CHAPTER 8

Vital energy

For people with severe respiratory conditions it is important to consider the emotional effects of the problem. We can survive for a considerable time without food and for several days without water, but only for a few minutes without breathing. If someone has breathing difficulties they feel, understandably, fearful and tense. Deep breathing exercises can address the problem both emotionally and physically. The exercises themselves, via the action of the diaphragm, massage the lungs and improve the circulation. There is a positive effect on the nervous system, with a reversal of the stress response, and the body being taken from the sympathetic into the parasympathetic state. Psychologically, the benefits can be huge, with the client being aware of a real sense of self-control, with no external intervention.

It can also be helpful to pay attention to clients' posture and to gently guide them, with hands-on support, to sit tall with relaxed, wide shoulders. Sometimes people with restricted breathing unconsciously adopt a self-protective stance of rounded shoulders, without being aware that it has happened. This reduces the lung capacity still further but, by simply correcting posture, breathing can be improved. Also, emotionally, spirits can be raised by sitting tall and confidently looking forward.

The reflex areas for the respiratory system are shown in *Figure 8.1*. The associated link is:

• Any tender lung area linked across to the spine.

For this link, any tender point which is found on the lung area, on either the plantar or dorsal aspect, is held with the thumb of one hand and then the other thumb is taken directly across to the spinal reflex on the medial line (see *Figure 8.2*).

Often heat is felt by the client, either on the reflex or in the actual lungs. Taking the tenderness across to the nerve intervention on the spine seems to relax the affected area, improving circulation and releasing tension.

The lungs in general are worked by applying pressure down the centre of the lung reflex area (both dorsal and plantar) and then spreading out the thumbs to each side of the foot. This creates a feeling of expansion and often encourages the client to breathe deeper.

The respiratory system is one of the body's eliminatory mechanisms. If there are respiratory problems there can also be tenderness in the digestive

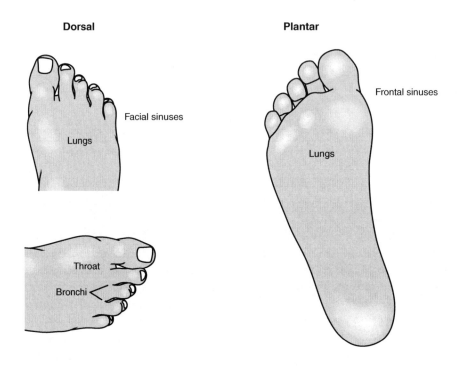

Figure 8.1: Reflexes for the respiratory system.

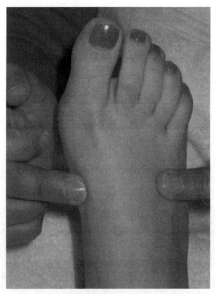

Figure 8.2: The lung to spine link.

reflex areas, this being another way in which the body eliminates toxins. Reflexology working on either of these two systems can indirectly benefit the other.

As a client relaxes during a treatment, breathing patterns noticeably change, becoming deeper and calmer. This provides an internal massage to the entire viscera. Depending on the nature of the client, and to restore a sense of balance, it can be very beneficial to advise either calming, or energising, breathing techniques depending on which are needed.

Case studies

I. Client details – Christine. Age 49.
Headteacher of a large school. Obviously this is a responsible position with high stress levels. She enjoys the job but often feels stressed and, because she has to work most evenings and some week-ends, she usually feels very tired.

Presenting symptom: Chronic painful sinusitis.
Treatment: On presentation the whole of the sinus reflexes were very tender. The pituitary and parathyroid areas were also painful. The ileo-caecal valve reflex was tender and felt hot to touch.

After four weekly treatments, the client reported having a very runny nose for two days and then being aware of noticeably reduced congestion, in her words "the best for a long time". After this the practitioner was able to apply stronger pressure as the sinus reflexes became less tender. At this time the client was also advised to reduce her intake of dairy food because of their mucous-forming properties and after the sixth treatment there were just isolated tender sinus points.

The treatments were reduced to monthly sessions and, after a further three sessions, the reflexes were completely free, as were the actual sinuses. It was discussed at this time, because the original presenting symptom had now been addressed, that she may want to discontinue treatment, just returning as and when necessary. However, Christine felt that because the treatment had helped in other ways, namely reducing stress levels and improving overall immunity, she would like to continue on a monthly basis. She maintains that she "needs to be given permission to switch off".

Incidentally, she was concerned about her weight gain and, after several months into the course of treatment, she said, "After all this attention, the least I can do is to look after myself" so she joined a local exercise class, reduced her food intake and took time to stop and eat lunch each day. She now has her weight under control.

2. Client details – James. Age 44.
Married with two teenage children. Computer technician.

Presenting symptom: Bronchitis. He had never experienced this before. He looked pale, tired and drawn.
Treatment: Several points over the lung area felt tender and each of these was linked across to the spinal reflex. Each time both points felt hot for the practitioner. James was guided through simple breathing exercises. His shoulder

areas were tight and tender and particular attention was given to the lymphatic system with a view to assisting the body's protective mechanism. James relaxed during the treatment and his breathing eased.

He received four-weekly treatments during the acute stage of his condition as he found this whole illness experience painful and frightening and wanted to make sure it didn't happen again. So, as a preventative measure, and because he enjoys them, he continues to practise deep breathing exercises at home, guided by a relaxation tape.

CHAPTER 9

Nourishment

The function of this system is to transport nourishment around to every part of the body. When a person feels cold and tired, either physically or emotionally, it can be a sign that the circulation is sluggish. Every part of the body needs an effective blood supply for correct functioning and, as circulation benefits enormously from movement, clients can help themselves with the introduction of appropriate exercise into their lifestyle.

Reflexology directly connects with the body's circulation touching the extremities of this all-important system on the hands and the feet. In traditional Chinese medicine the quality of the blood and circulation is a primary diagnostic sign of health and illness. The Nei Ching, a text on ancient Chinese medicine, states that the pulse can be,

"...sharp as a hook, fine as a hair, taut as a musical string, dead as a rock, smooth as a flowing stream or as continuous as a string of pearls." (Majno, 1975)

It is interesting to note that these words quite accurately describe the sensitive responses often felt during reflexology treatment. Much more accurately, in fact, than Western words, which often seem to be too analytical and measured.

During a standard full reflexology treatment the whole of the body's circulation is stimulated and improved. The specific link for the circulatory system is:

- Adrenal reflex linked to the groin reflex.

This link is located by holding the adrenal reflex with the thumb of one hand and, with the middle finger of each hand, connecting to the groin reflexes (see *Figure 9.1*).

This link can feel powerful with a sense of connection between the points and often heat is felt on the adrenal reflex area. It can be especially beneficial for clients with sluggish

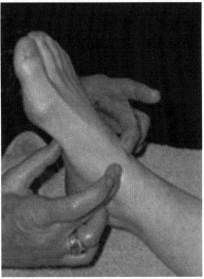

Figure 9.1: The adrenal to groin link.

circulation, having a stimulating effect. It also appears to be beneficial as an added "boost" for the adrenal gland in helping to restore salt and water balance in cases of fluid retention.

Case studies

1. Client details – Harry. Age 67.
Widower. Retired.

Presenting symptom: Diabetic. Harry manages this condition well but is concerned about the poor circulation in his feet.

Treatment: On presentation his feet are pale and extremely cold to touch. They became pinker and warmer in response to foot massage. During the treatment the adrenal to groin link was held several times on each foot. The adrenal point felt very tender – in fact, he instinctively pulled his foot away – so a light touch was used.

He received regular monthly treatments and, after the third one, he reported that his feet felt warmer and that they stayed warmer for longer periods of time. This had remained so, with monthly treatments in the winter and bi-monthly ones in the summer. His toes usually feel numb initially but warm up during the session. His poor circulation can still be a problem in the winter, but there has been no worsening of the situation despite his diabetes. During the consultation he often talks fondly about his late wife. He is obviously lonely and misses her terribly; he doesn't become upset but seems to enjoy the opportunity to reminisce.

2. Client details – Audrey. Age 52.
After a long history of spinal problems, she had surgery several years ago which resulted in fusion of the lumbar vertebrae. She is realistic about her limitations and manages to have a full and active life. Married with three grown up children.

Presenting symptom: Poor circulation and night-time cramps in her legs.
Treatment: She receives regular monthly treatments. After the second session she reported that the cramps were less frequent. She is very responsive throughout the treatment. Whenever the pituitary reflex is worked she feels a slight pulsing sensation in her temples; when the lumbar 5 to hip link is held she feels a "floating and heavy sensation, as though waves are passing over" her. At the same time, the practitioner feels a charge of energy through her own arms. The adrenal to groin link often produces slight palpitations in

Audrey's chest which feel strange but not unpleasant; she breathes deeply and the feeling subsides.

After the fourth treatment, Audrey said that her feet and legs were warmer and the cramp was much improved, with some nights being totally free. Two months later she was thrilled, saying that her feet were now warmer than her husband's, and her overall circulation has improved. She has regular treatments at six-weekly intervals and the improvement has been sustained.

Recently, as she greeted the practitioner, she announced proudly, "I feel so good about myself."

Reference

Majno G (1975) *The Healing Hand: Man and Wound in the Ancient World*. Cambridge MA, Harvard University Press: 245

CHAPTER 10

Reproduction

This sensitive system, perhaps more than any other, reflects inevitable life changes whether these be physical, emotional, social or cultural. This area of the body may alter the way that it has previously functioned, as though it mirrors the associated emotions presented by the new, challenging situation. The reflexes for the reproductive system are shown in *Figure 10.1*.

The links associated with this system are:
• Ovary to uterus
• Ovary to uterus to pituitary gland.

To locate the ovary to uterus link, hold the uterus reflex on the medial aspect of the foot with the middle finger of one hand and the ovary reflex on the lateral aspect with the middle finger of the other hand (see *Figure 10.2*). The ovary reflex can be held still while the uterus is worked with circular thumb pressure.

In order to reinforce the natural process within the endocrine system, this two-way link can be connected to the pituitary gland reflex point. To do this, the middle finger stays on the ovary reflex but now the thumb of the same hand holds the uterus so that the other thumb can locate the pituitary reflex point as in *Figure 10.3*.

These links can obviously be used for any problems with menstruation. The three-way link is particularly effective for any conditions involving irregularity in the menstrual cycle, for helping to restore a sense of balance and, also, for conditions associated with stress. Taking into account contraindications (see Chapter 13), these links should not be used during pregnancy.

Both these links often feel soft and delicate; a light touch being particularly appropriate. Vibrations can be felt through the foot, or, with the three-way link, contained within a triangle of energy around the pelvic area reflexes. Interestingly, especially for this particular system, clients report a feeling of being held or cradled. This also supports the emotional state that often accompanies any disorders of this system.

The manner in which a person is not well, ie. the presenting symptom, often reflects how the person is feeling emotionally, and conditions affecting the reproductive system are no exception to this. It seems to be no coincidence that the menopause, commonly referred to as "the change", when a woman's reproductive cycle begins to alter, happens at a time

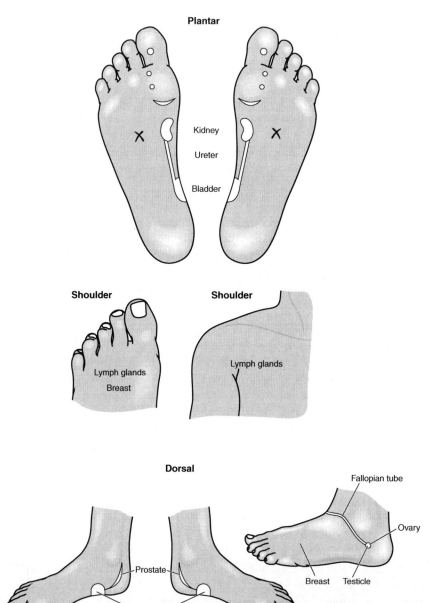

Figure 10.1: Reflexes for the reproductive system.

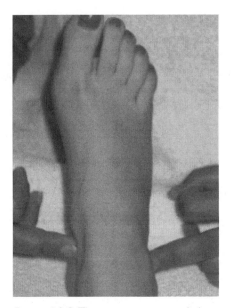

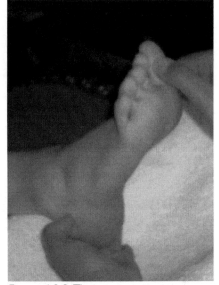

Figure 10.2: The ovary to uterus link.

Figure 10.3: The ovary to uterus to pituitary link.

of major lifestyle developments such as children leaving home, parents becoming dependant and possible career moves. These situations are not necessarily better or worse but certainly they are different and challenging and, inevitably, they call for emotional changes. Often an awareness of this connection between symptoms, emotions and lifestyle, creates a positive situation which supports a natural progression. There can be less emphasis on individual symptoms and more on a positive approach involving self-help and support mechanisms at a time of great transition.

Case study

Client details – Alison. Age 28.
Married. No children but she and her husband are wanting to start a family. Nurse.

Presenting symptom: Irritable bowel syndrome (IBS). Alison experiences spells of abdominal bloating and diarrhoea. She has endometriosis which has only been diagnosed recently; over the last six months she has had heavy and painful periods. She often feels tired.

Treatment: On presentation there was a high degree of tension in the neck reflex, a very strong reaction on the pituitary gland reflex and the right ovary reflex point was very sensitive. The reflexes for the small and large intestines felt tight on both feet. Alison received a full treatment, the aim being to reduce overall stress levels and special attention was given to the endocrine system in an attempt to restore homeostasis. She fell asleep quickly but this appeared to be due to tiredness rather than relaxation.

At the first two sessions, the ovary to uterus link was held lightly, the vibrations on the two points felt out of balance to the practitioner and the client felt heat on the ovary reflex point. Thereafter, this was converted into the three-way link by also holding the pituitary gland reflex. The sensation of heat on the ovary was reduced and Alison described "a pulse feeling moving between the three points".

After four fortnightly appointments, the neck tension was considerably reduced, the overall response was calmer and her periods have, in her words, "settled down". The intestinal reflexes feel softer and she appears to be free of the IBS symptoms. After a further three monthly treatments, her menstrual cycle has reverted back to how it was before the endometriosis was diagnosed. She is noticeably calmer, brighter and more relaxed generally. Since starting the course of treatment she has begun to attend a weekly Yoga class.

Note: the client at this time became pregnant. She continued with the Yoga classes but not with reflexology due to work commitments. She and her husband now have a beautiful baby daughter.

CHAPTER 11

Protection

The lymphatic system has a cleansing and protecting effect on the body. When it is struggling it is a true case of lack of harmony with the environment, either internally within the body or externally with the world. Clients report feeling vulnerable and they use phrases such as, "If there is an infection around then I'll get it." Reassurance and a positive attitude within the dialogue of the consultation are often valuable in themselves.

Reflexology, with its direct contact with some of the lymphatic structures of the body, can have a powerful effect on this system. Care should be taken not to detoxify a highly toxic person too quickly, but rather to do this gradually in an acceptable way that can be maintained.

Practical, realistic changes to diet and exercise can improve lymphatic function and increase the body's protection. Also, this self-help approach can promote feelings of being empowered and lift a person's spirits. Dietary recommendations involve receiving energy and protection from fresh, whole, untreated foods (see Chapter 14).

The lymphatic fluid requires movement in order to be able to travel through the body. Therefore, exercise, in ways that are realistic, appropriate and enjoyable for each individual, is vital.

The movement of lymphatic fluid that can result from a reflexology treatment is reflected in the way that recipients often describe themselves as feeling "lighter" after such a treatment.

The specific reflexes for the lymphatic system are shown in *Figure 11.1*. But also, during a full treatment, the function of the lymph system is inevitably improved by the direct action of any foot massage strokes that are included in the procedure.

The specific link for this system is:
• The thymus gland is linked to itself.

This is achieved by holding the thymus reflex (on the plantar aspect of each foot) with one thumb and then, with the middle of the other hand, holding a point immediately above on the dorsal aspect (see *Figure 11.2*). Often heat is felt, with a sense of connection through the foot. Alternatively, if a person's immune system is compromised, then it can feel flat and lifeless. In this way this link can be used to boost immunity if it is appropriate to do so. At times of stress it can be helpful to give the thymus added attention; this gland has a vital role in that it matures "T" cells (these form part of the

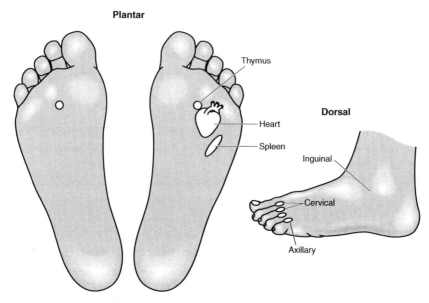

Figure 11.1: Reflexes for the lymphatic system.

body's immune processes) and this function is impaired when the body is under stress.

When the lymph system is sluggish, resulting in fluid retention, it can be beneficial to give extra attention to the urinary system during treatment. This can involve using the pituitary to adrenal link referred to in Chapter 7. As an addition to this link, the pituitary remains held while working down from the adrenal gland reflex to the urether onto the bladder reflexes, then back to the adrenal gland. This appears to assist the body in restoring its salt/water balance.

Within a treatment, the most effective way of improving lymphatic function is with effleurage massage strokes, working towards the heart. The lymphatic system can become sluggish for a variety of reasons, including illness, injury, trauma, poor nutrition, the effect of pollution, lack of exercise, medication, infection or stress. It has been proven that stress directly affects the body's level of immunity. In the 1980s Drs Jan and Ron Glaser, in America, conducted studies to find out if stress could have any effect on the cells of the immune system (Glaser and Glaser 1987). They set up a control experience using a group of medical students and measured the activity of white blood cells; key cells of the body's defence against disease. They found out that, immediately after taking exams, the students had less active white blood cells. The Glasers also conducted a detailed study on carers with relatives who have Alzheimer's disease to monitor the effect on health of continuous, long-term stress. The findings showed that in these people the immune response was lowered; the wounds of over-stressed carers took 24% longer to heal than did those of unstressed people. As a result of its ability to promote relaxation, it can be seen that reflexology will have a positive effect on the immune system.

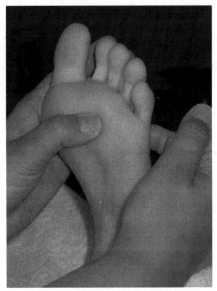

Figure 11.2: The thymus link.

Case study

Client details – Jean. Age 39. Married with two small sons.

Presenting symptoms: Fluid retention. Puffy hands and feet pre-menstrually. This can be so severe at times that Jean says her fingers look like "sausages", she cannot bend them and, sometimes, cannot even pick up a cup. Underactive thyroid gland. Overweight. She feels heavy and weighty.

Treatment: She received a full treatment with particular attention to lymphatic drainage and to the reflexes of the thyroid gland. All the lymphatic reflexes were very tender to touch and so very light effleurage strokes were used; the reflexes for the entire endocrine system were also very painful to touch. The thyroid link to itself was used; this felt very tingly to the practitioner and to Jean it felt very warm and it ached. The thymus link felt flat and lifeless. Throughout the treatment, effleurage strokes were repeated to help drain the lymphatic fluid.

At the first session Jean enjoyed the time to focus on herself and to talk about her concerns regarding her weight. She knows that she lacks the time and the motivation to exercise and diet. Immediately after the treatment, and all subsequent ones, she needed to rush to the toilet. After the initial three weekly appointments, she reported frequent urination for the following twenty-four hours and extreme tiredness. During this time she had a period and was amazed that she had no fluid retention. She has not lost any weight but feels "lighter".

The treatments were reduced to fortnightly for a further two months. The tiredness after the sessions ceased and the fluid retention became minimal. The thymus link now felt energetic. This remains the case, except when Jean is tired or stressed and then the link is held for a longer time until the energetic vibration is felt. She now felt ready to address the weight problem. She and the practitioner discussed a diet which would fit in with her lifestyle and activity levels. She also joined a local gym.

The treatments are now at monthly intervals, she feels supported by the consultations and reports back with progress of her weight loss. Nine months after the first session, she said, "I can now look at myself in the mirror without cringing." She continues with regular treatments, with occasional problems with fluid retention but these are easily corrected. She continues to enjoy the "time-out".

References

Glaser J, Glaser R. (1987) Chronic Stress and Immunity in family caregivers of Alzheimer's disease victims. Psychosomatic Medicine .Vol.49:523-535.

CHAPTER 12

Sensations

Our senses are the way in which we absorb information from our environment for interpretation. Understandably, if this is restricted in any way, then we feel isolated, vulnerable, depressed and often frightened. The reflexology consultation provides an ideal forum in which to offer support and reassurance. The reflexes for these areas are delicate and sensitive, as are the organs themselves, therefore the touch required needs to be equally light, sensitive and reassuring. There are no specific reflexes for the vital sense of touch but, obviously, this receives direct benefits during a treatment and, indirectly, by the positive effect on the entire nervous system.

The therapeutic benefits of touch, physiological and emotional, cannot be underestimated in the context of a reflexology treatment.

"The greatest sense in our body is our touch sense. It is probably the chief sense in the processes of sleeping and waking; it gives us our knowledge of depth or thickness and form; we feel, we love and hate, are touchy and are touched, through the touch corpuscles of our skin."
J.Lionel Taylor, 1921

When we are born, touch is our most heightened sense, it is our first form of communication, being beyond words. Bertrand Russell said, "... our whole conception of what exists outside us, is based on the sense of touch." To be cared for and touched is a basic human need and vital for the healthy development of each individual. Ashley Montagu (1986) in his book "Touching" says,

"By being stroked and caressed, and carried, and cuddled, comforted, and cooed to, by being loved, the child learns to stroke and caress and cuddle, comfort and coo, and to love others."

Tiffany Field, at the Touch Research Institute in Miami, conducted extensive studies (1986) into the value of touch, in particular for premature babies. These studies show how, with regular massage, premature babies had a greater weight gain than babies who were not massaged. Perhaps, more importantly, this improvement in development was still evident when the babies reached one year old.

In Sweden, the Axelsons Gymastiska Institut (1998) has conducted studies with children. After integrating massage into the daily routine in more than one thousand kindergartens, the children became calmer, could concentrate more easily and were more sociable in groups.

Touching is often not a part of daily life in Western cultures and sometimes it highlights inhibitions and even taboos in certain situations. With reflexology, clients can receive a "safe" and appropriate touch which, in itself, can have a beneficially therapeutic effect.

The skin can often reflect emotions, for example we blush with embarrassment. Tension and stress can present themselves in the form of skin conditions such as eczema and psoriasis. Often the words that someone uses to describe their skin problem also matches their emotional state, for example someone who is frustrated and restricted may say their skin is "breaking out", as though that is the only breaking out that they are capable of at that time.

The reflex areas for the sensory organs and associated areas are shown in *Figure 12.1*.

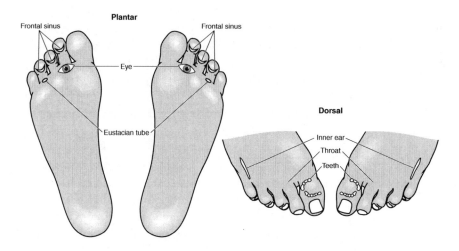

Figure 12.1: Reflexes for the sensory organs.

Case studies

1. Client details – Emma. Age 47.
Married with no children. Senior clerical officer. There have been redundancies at work and, while her own job appears to be secure, she has now an increased work load with fewer staff.

Presenting symptoms: Chronic tinnitus. Emma has had this problem for ten years. It is aggravated by stress and at present it is very evident and constant. She is inevitably depressed because of this. She finds it difficult to concentrate and is exhausted, both physically and mentally.

She is very familiar with this long-term condition and has realistic expectations of the treatment outcome. She would like to achieve a reduction in the symptoms so that it feels manageable to her again. She is very aware of the effect of stress on her overall health in general and on the tinnitus in particular.

Treatment: On presentation the pituitary, forebrain and neck reflexes were all tender and tense. Relevant links were used, ie. forebrain to sacrum, pituitary to adrenal and neck to jaw. The inner ear reflexes were extremely sensitive, especially on the left foot. These were worked lightly and returned to several times during treatment. The practitioner showed Emma the inner ear reflex points on her hands so she could work these points herself between the sessions. She found this helpful and was able to monitor the condition by the degree of sensitivity.

Immediately after each treatment the tinnitus was very noisy for two days and then became much quieter for varying lengths of time; sometimes this improvement lasts for one week and sometimes for as long as two weeks, the extent of the benefit appearing to match her stress levels.

After the third treatment, Emma began to relax during the session. She enjoys this now, looks forward to it and feels that it helps her to cope with the stresses of her job better than before. The neck and jaw area is always tender and she realises exactly how much tension she can hold in that area; often she was so tense that when she woke up in the morning her jaw was clenched. The reflexology has made her aware of this, so she practises some simple relaxation techniques before going to sleep and this seems to be reducing the tension.

2. Client details – Elsie. Age 54.
Married. One adult daughter. She is very self-conscious, timid and frequently apologises for herself for no apparent reason. She works as a secretary.

Presenting symptom: High blood pressure. Elsie says that this frightens her. She talks a lot and, again, apologises for this, saying it is because she is nervous. Often she talks about situations in her life when she has missed opportunities because she was afraid to take a risk and she seems to be generally fearful.

Treatment: At the first session she was nervous and anxious. This was mainly a foot massage treatment with lots of reassurance. She was obviously unhappy with her working situation and described her job as "the general skivvy"; she felt that she was given work that no-one else would do. However, she also accepted that this was often her own fault because she didn't speak up for herself and just accepted what was given to her. Her feet were extremely tense.

As the course of treatment progressed she relaxed and more reflexology techniques could be used to replace the massage. The neck and shoulder reflexes were always tight and tender initially but they both relaxed during treatment. The thyroid link was very powerful and felt slightly uncomfortable for her. Also the throat reflex area was tender and she did in fact have frequent throat infections. It was as though this was reflecting her ability to communicate and she said that she found it difficult to express herself.

Over a period of six months she changed in appearance, looking more confident and smiling more often. She quietly became more confident at work, being able to tell her immediate superior how she felt and she was much happier as a result. She still had the same apologetic manner but relaxed and enjoyed the treatments more. For relaxation at home and to help her feel more empowered she was guided through a basic breathing and relaxation exercise. She found that this also helped her when she was bottling up her feelings. Her blood pressure went down slightly and she was less anxious about this. In addition, she had fewer throat infections.

References

Axelsons Gymnastiska Institut (1998) Box 6475, 11382 Stockholm

Field T (1986) Touch Research Institute University of Miami, School of Medicine, PO Box 016820, Miami, FL33101, USA

Montagu A (1986) *Touching*. Harper and Row, USA: 126

Taylor JL (1921) The Stages of Human Life. In Montagu A (1986) *Touching*. Harper and Row, New York: 3

CHAPTER 13

Precision reflexology: Procedure and charts

"Linking" is one technique, forming part of a full reflexology treatment. The precision reflexology chart (see *Figure 13.1*) is used as a "map" to cover the whole of the body.

Hand treatments can also be used, see *Figure 13.2*. Hand reflexology can be given if the feet are inaccessible for any reason, for instance in cases of severe injury or infection. Occasionally it is a client's preference. Working on hands is an invaluable form of reinforcement between sessions and a genuine way to establish the principle of self-help.

The main stroke used within treatments is a slow rotating thumb pressure, interspersed with effleurage and percussion massage strokes. It is always beneficial to commence a treatment with a general foot massage sequence (including mobilisation of the foot and ankle) so as to reassure clients, to give them time to settle down, to introduce an element of relaxation and for the practitioner to begin to assess the level of stress within each person.

The overall procedure is outlined in the chart shown in *Figure 13.3* with links being integrated in the relevant areas. This is obviously a standard, general treatment which would be adapted to suit each individual, with more or less emphasis on certain areas. The practitioner is guided by the sensitivity in his/her hands, by intuition, by the client's responses and by a holistic knowledge of the anatomy and physiology of the body.

As with all massage, there are a variety of strokes that can be adapted, the overall principle being that the client should feel at times interested, curious, involved, or relaxed but always secure, with a sense of being held safely.

Generally, the deeper the stroke, the more effective it will be (except for linking when a light touch is always required). Tenderness usually indicates an imbalance so the pressure used should always be within comfortable limits. If clients receiving a treatment are constantly fearful and anticipating pain then they cannot, consciously or unconsciously, allow themselves to heal. The aim is for the body to be in a relaxed, parasympathetic state. On tender areas it is more effective to apply comfortable pressure and then to return to the same reflex several times during the treatment (and in subsequent treatments), each time being able to use slightly more pressure.

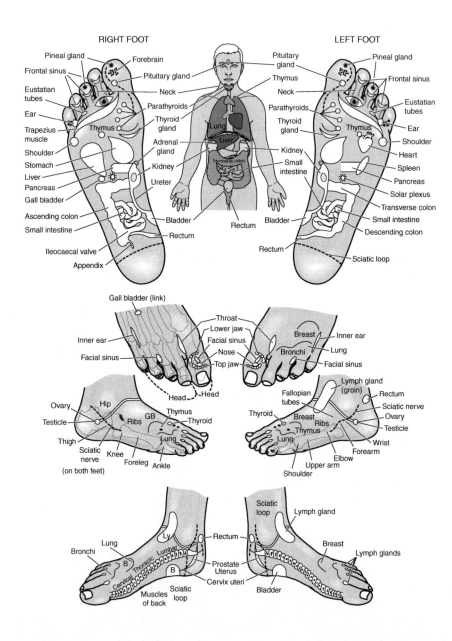

Figure 13.1: Precision reflexology chart.

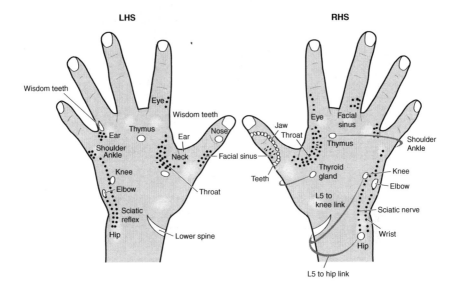

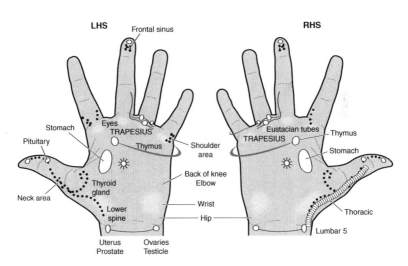

Figure 13.2: Hand chart.

Relaxation massage to begin - on both feet.

Right foot:	Left foot:
Solar plexus	Solar plexus
Thyroid gland L	Thyroid L
Parathyroid glands L	Parathyroid glands L
Neck L	Neck L
Pituitary gland L	Pituitary gland L
Forebrain L	Forebrain L
Pineal gland L	Pineal gland L
Sinuses	Sinuses
Throat	Throat
Eyes	Eyes
Eustacian tubes	Eustacian tubes
Ears	Ears
Bronchi	Bronchi
Lungs – dorsal and plantar aspects of foot L	Lungs – dorsal/plantar aspects of foot L
Lymph area – dorsal	Lymph – dorsal
Breast	Breast
Shoulders L	Shoulders L
Thymus L	Thymus L
Diaphragm	Diaphragm
Liver	Heart
Gall bladder L	Stomach
Stomach	Spleen
Small intestines	Pancreas
Ascending colon	Small intestines
1st half of transverse colon	2nd half of transverse colon
Kidney	Descending colon
Adrenal gland L	Sigmoid colon to rectum
Ureter to bladder	Kidney
Muscles of spine	Adrenal gland L
Spine L	Ureter to bladder
Leg L	Muscles of spine
Arm L	Spine L
Reproductive system L	Leg L
Lymph – back of heel	Arm L

Right foot:	Left foot:
Effleurage	Reproductive system L
	Lymph – back of heel
	Effleurage

Finishing with a reassuring hold of both feet to accompany the client's deep breathing.

N.B. "L" indicates where a link can be used if appropriate.

Figure 13.3: Precision reflexology procedure.

In this way, the body can heal in its own time gradually and effectively, without force. The linking technique of precision work is especially helpful on tender reflexes because the treatment can be energetic with a very light touch. A parallel principle here is captured in the Chinese saying that the quickest way from A to B is not in a direct line (see *Figure 13.4*) as this can be too forceful, so will be met with resistance and, thus, rejected. Rather, the most efficient way could be to take a softer approach which can be readily accepted. There is also a Yogic principle which maintains that it is possible to be strong and relaxed at the same time. This says that control and tension are not synonymous. It is possible to achieve a state of balance with both steadiness (in Sanskrit this is called Stkira) and relaxation (in Sanskrit this is Sukha) present together (see *Figure 13.5*). Similarities with this Yogic philosophy and the application of reflexology can be seen in the combination both of firm and gentle massage strokes.

If we accept that the feet represent the energy of the body, then each reflex area needs to be handled in an appropriate way. Firmer pressure can be applied to the more robust areas, eg. the shoulders, and a lighter touch to the more delicate structures, eg. the eyes. Also, receiving the treatment will feel different for different points, eg. the areas relating to the intestines tend

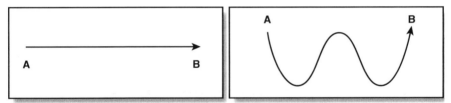

Figure 13.4: Effective soft approach.

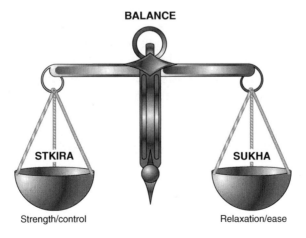

Figure 13.5: Balance of Sukha and Stkira.

to produce dull, bruised reactions and the neurological areas invoke sharp and tingling sensations.

There is an endless variety of reactions that can be felt by the practitioner. For instance, the reflexes can feel crystalline, bubbly, fibrous, hot, cold, soft or tense. Also there are less tangible responses which have been described using words such as energetic, lethargic, sharp, dull, empty and full. The sensitive practitioner can decipher this information, and relate it to the particular organ and to the nature of each client, in order to establish if it is appropriate or not.

Client reactions differ, some feeling responses in the feet only, with others having sensations in the related body part. Both are equally valid – reflecting how that person is functioning at that time.

Improvements in health are rarely steady and consistent but usually progress with natural fluctuations, reflecting the "ups and downs" that clients report. Thankfully, this sequence of events often results in the benefits being sustained. The power of the healing needs to be in the client's own time and own way and not as a result of the will or ego of the practitioner.

Experienced practitioners can "translate" the reactions that are felt through the fingers into a therapeutic understanding of the client. For instance, when working the solar plexus reflex then the pressure used needs to feel positive and acceptable, but not painful. Reactions differ from person to person and from treatment to treatment. Often the reality of the response is quite different from the external presentation of the person; this reflex point may feel sensitive and vulnerable or, indeed, robust and energetic, either state often indicating a quite different persona from the one that the client presents.

The pressure used is matched to the health, sensitivity and nature of each part of the body. For example, no caring person would apply strong pressure to the top of someone's head, therefore light touch is applied to the reflex for the top of the head situated at the top of each toe. In the same way, the reflexology pressure used on the reflexes for the large muscles of the shoulders will differ considerably from that used on delicate structures such as the sinus points. Likewise, a healthy liver is a robust organ so a deep pressure can be used on its reflex point whereas a lighter touch would be appropriate for the reflexes for the more fragile kidneys.

The consultation situation aims to be, at times, pleasurable and relaxing and, at other times, challenging and provocative, while always being constructive and positive.

General guidelines for the "linking" technique

There are few times when reflexology would not be recommended but, as each treatment is adapted to the individual recipient, there may be situations when caution is needed. General, overall guidelines are shown in the box below with contraindications listed on page 72.

Please note that precision reflexology is now widely used in the care of cancer patients at Christie's Hospital in Manchester (Mackereth and Carter 2006).

These are general guidelines and each situation must be considered in its own right. An important principle is that the practitioner and the client/patient must both feel confident to proceed with the treatment.

Guidelines for "linking" techniques

- The responses are a reflection of the subtle energy levels of each client and, as such, they won't necessarily be obvious and vibrant
- Responses differ from one person to another and from treatment to treatment, the ideal situation being for the energy to match the nature of the recipient.
- The application is a non-judgemental acceptance of how that person is functioning at that time.
- Whatever is felt is a true and correct feeling, operating on an instinctive level, and it is beyond words.
- It is advisable not to work all the links within each session but, instead, to be selective, using ones that are appropriate for the client's needs.
- Generally speaking, the stronger the reaction then the more effective the link will be.
- If possible, hold the link until a change in vibration is felt.
- Trust the intuition response.

Contraindications to precision reflexology

• Conditions such as deep vein thrombosis or phlebitis, which would not respond favourably to stimulation, should not be treated.
• Patients taking regular medication, such as thyroxin or insulin, should be made aware that reflexology can positively affect these conditions so that they need to monitor themselves in case an adjustment of medication is required.
• During pregnancy it is advisable to avoid treatment for the first thirteen weeks until the pregnancy is established. Thereafter, as a precautionary measure, do not work the reproductive or pituitary gland reflexes. Extreme caution is needed if the woman has a history of unstable pregnancies.
• Clients with heart conditions can be treated with the recommendation of their doctor. Obviously, the heart reflex point itself is avoided. In these cases stress is often a considerable factor so the relaxation achieved during a treatment has a positive effect.
• Cancer patients in general will benefit from the treatment. However, because of the effect on the immune system, it is advisable not to treat if the patient is receiving chemotherapy or radiotherapy. Obviously the reflex for the area where the cancer has occurred should be avoided. In terminal cases, the positive effect of touch and tender loving care cannot be underestimated.

Reference

Mackereth P, Carter A (2006). *Massage and Bodywork – adapting therapies for cancer care*. Churchill Livingstone, Edinburgh: 210

CHAPTER 14

Complete holistic healthcare

Complementary health practitioners share an overriding ethos within their work, and this has two major aims:

- To restore a state of homeostasis to the health of each client
- To encourage each client to begin to take responsibility for his/her own health.

Each therapy uses its own particular approach to try to achieve these aims but also, in order to maintain the benefits over a period of time, it is essential to consider how each individual can look after him/herself. Surely what really matters is what happens in the interval between the consultations. The truly important aspect of each person's health status must surely be how he/she can restore, and realistically maintain health and well-being. Each person is able to do this in varying degrees depending on age, lifestyle, personal preference and overall state of health. Obviously reflexologists use their own techniques to achieve this situation but we cannot underestimate the value of self-help; the ultimate power is in the hands of the client/patient. The self-esteem from this empowerment has, in turn, a positive effect on health (see *Figure 14.1*).

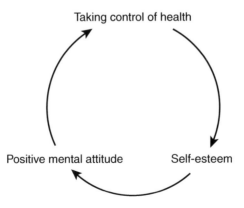

Taking control of health

Positive mental attitude   Self-esteem

Figure 14.1: The positive effect of self-help.

The consultation often acts as a catalyst to "trigger" motivation for the client to act. Hopefully, as clients begin to ask themselves, "How am I to-day?" and "How do I feel?", the next question will be "What can I do about it?". Each person needs strategies or life skills to apply to this increased self-awareness. Ideally, any changes need to be manageable, gradual and certainly not a cause of stress in themselves. The steps taken need to feel realistic; in this way they can become an acceptable and enjoyable part of life.

Ways of achieving self-care

Diet and nutrition: the aim is to receive energy from food and to eat with enjoyment in a relaxed, sociable manner. The guidelines for each person need to be feasible, even if challenging, as any sense of resentment or denial will lead to tension and a sense of imbalance. The most appropriate dictum is to aim for food that has been treated as little as possible. Modern food production with techniques such as genetic engineering and the extensive use of pesticides, presents obstacles to be overcome. The intake of "non-foods" such as sugar and salt, and stimulants such as coffee, alcohol and nicotine should be avoided or, at least, reduced. There may be specific advice for some health problems, for instance to reduce acid-forming foods in cases of arthritis, to reduce dairy foods for some respiratory problems or to increase the intake of fresh, organic fruit and vegetables in order to boost immunity.

There is always an emotional element with food; how and what we eat is the ultimate expression of our self-care. The reflexology consultation can perhaps begin to address these issues as the client/practitioner relationship develops.

Exercise: energy is movement. Obviously this needs to be matched to the ability, lifestyle and temperament of each person. An equal sense of achievement can be obtained for one person by completing a six-mile run and, for another, by walking to the garden gate. Again the principle should be one of enjoyment. This may be a specific exercise for a particular problem, for instance to reduce congestion and pain during menstruation, or a routine for general fitness. The sense of well-being achieved by regular exercise has a positive effect on all levels; the physical benefits are obvious, stress is reduced and the spirits are restored by the release of the body's own natural relaxant, the endorphins.

Relaxation: to achieve some exclusive time for oneself breaks the stress response and has a positive effect physically, mentally and spiritually. This may be of a certain design, for example Yoga or Tai Chi, or it may be creating a few quiet moments within the day, such as going for a walk in the countryside. Being surrounded by beautiful scenery, feeling a part of nature reaffirms the Oriental belief that each human spirit is a part of the wider universe.

The body is designed to cope with short-term stress; damage occurs if this becomes constant and long-term. This situation depletes the body's energy whether it be on a physical, emotional or spiritual level. Relaxation with conscious awareness not only prevents the accumulation of stress, but also increases self-awareness of how it feels to be relaxed in contrast to how it feels to be stressed. Often stress has a gradual build-up over a period of time and relaxation provides a way of standing back to review the situation. Stress can be seen as a response to change, accompanied by a feeling of loss of control. Involvement with one's own healthcare can help to counter these feelings. Energy levels can be restored so that, with increased vitality and clarity of mind, the individual can function in a more efficient and self-contained manner. Leonardo da Vinci said,

"Every now and then go away, have a little relaxation, for when you come back to your work your judgement will be surer; since to remain constantly at work will cause you to lose power of judgement. Go some distance away because the work appears smaller and more of it can be taken in at a glance, and a lack of harmony or proportion is more readily seen."

Does this last sentence refer to life or art, or both? Often success and stress are thought to be synonymous. The Yogic principle mentioned in Chapter 13 demonstrates that strength and control (stkira) can exist side-by-side with relaxation and ease (sukha), in fact the one can ideally be balanced by the other. Complementary therapy acknowledges the unique nature of each individual, this is evident in the approach to stress; what is stressful to one person is simply healthy motivation to another. Equally, what may seem like a trivial situation to one person, to another would present a major opportunity for stress and tension. Within a consultation each individual response is obviously respected as being how that person functions. Just as unique is the manner of relaxation; some prefer a set, focused procedure with specific breathing techniques, while others achieve the same benefits by consciously creating some "time out".

"You cannot lead a balanced life without periods of relaxation. This is not the same as sleep, which is a combination of restfulness and specific internal activity. Relaxation is the vital process of letting-go." Howard Kent, 1993

Relaxation may sound gentle and soft, and this is so, but it can have a powerful effect.

Breathing: many people have become lazy in their manner of breathing. Often simple, deep breathing techniques can have a dramatic effect on energy levels. Deep breathing is simple and totally non-invasive. No special equipment is needed, neither is any external intervention. It acts as an internal massage, has a beneficial effect on every system of the body and restores a sense of calm. Specific breathing techniques can be matched to each individual and each situation. It may be appropriate to adopt slow, deep breathing to reduce tension and to help gain control in stressful situations or to practice energising breaths to counter tiredness. It can take quite a time to relinquish established patterns of breathing and to re-learn new ones.

How we breathe is often taken for granted but all stresses and strains will affect the flow of breath, so we can never afford to ignore it. Huge benefits are to be gained from being aware of the movement and value of each breath. A strong sense of self-control and self-management, that is both simple and powerful, can be achieved by being in charge of this vital process.

We can affect how we feel and function with how we breathe. In stressful situations, the vital instinctive response for the body is to breathe rapidly. The effect of slow, deep breathing is to reverse the stress response by sending calming messages around the body and mind to say that it is not a stressful situation. Specific visualisation methods, in conjunction with breathing patterns, can be used to help alleviate tension and pain.

"Breathe naturally, without forcing. No pressure, no disturbance, nothing should interfere with the simple, tide-like movement of our lungs as we breathe in and out." Vanda Scaravelli, 1991

Each of these modalities can be introduced into the consultation as and when the practitioner feels it appropriate – the skill being to know how much to introduce and when. This is a measure of the quality of each therapeutic relationship – so that clients feel empowered as well as secure and supported. This self-help approach is outlined in specific detail in connection with its role in advanced precision reflexology in Chapter 16.

Holistic foot care

Reflexologists believe that any imbalances within the system are reflected in the feet so it seems reasonable to believe that any problems with the feet themselves could be reflected in the body. It would also seem fair to accept that this is a two-way connection. Therefore a valuable form of self-help is to take good care of our feet. The most obvious and effective way of doing this is the selection of the shoes that we wear.

Badly fitting shoes can cause foot problems, such as bunions and corns (these can have an effect in reflexology terms on the related parts of the body) and impact on the structure of the body, especially the spine, by interfering with natural balance and alignment.

The body only needs to be slightly out of line, for instance a person may stand with more weight on one foot than on the other, and this, over the years, can result in chronic back pain as all structures of the body try to compensate. This can sometimes be corrected by being aware of the misalignment and by adjusting posture, or by exercises to strengthen the weaker area.

Often skeletal problems, particularly of the spine, pelvis and ankles can be alleviated by professional advice on foot mechanics. Such advice can provide support, reduce discomfort and also help to re-align the structures of the body. An example of this is a thirty-five year old woman who presented with acute lumbar spine pain. She received reflexology which gave her short term relief but, to provide long-term care, it was necessary to address the cause of the problem. She has always been knock-kneed and when she walked she swung her legs slightly out to the side with each step. She was referred to a local shoe-maker who also practised foot mechanics and he made her some shoes with specifically designed supports in the sole and the result was dramatic. Within weeks, her back problem had vanished and she could walk for long distances which had previously been impossible.

Shoes that are made to measure for each individual not only match the feet, but also, match the person and his or her unique body mechanics.

References

Kent H (1993) *The Complete Yoga Course*. Headline Book Publishing Ltd, London: 31

Scaravelli V (1991) *Awakening the Spine*. Harper Collins Publishers, London: 176

CHAPTER 15

Precision reflexology: A complementary therapy

The primary focus behind all complementary therapy is to care rather than to cure. Reflexology provides an opportunity for people to be cared for and, more importantly, to begin to care for themselves. It sets aside exclusive time which is valuable and healing in itself.

There is no one defined way to feel well or unwell and the symptoms that people describe are their own way of saying that they are not well. Each individual presents for treatment with a unique set of symptoms which reflect how they are functioning at that time, physically, emotionally and spiritually. Ideally, through the treatments, individuals can feel involved in their own healthcare and become aware of all the various aspects of life that contribute to their state of health. This sense of empowerment may be apparent in practical ways, represented by realistic and appropriate life-style changes. The effect of this self-help approach increases self-esteem, resulting in an increased sense of well-being. There may be less obvious changes as this involvement also provokes questions such as, "Why this problem and why at this time?" or "How does this make me feel?" or "Can the nature of this illness tell me anything?" The answers to question like these can demonstrate how the body reflects the emotions. The conscious realisation of this can then influence future healthcare (this concept is further explained in Chapter 16). Sometimes the emotional connection is easy to see, but sometimes it is not such an obvious attachment. It is important not to involve any sense of guilt or blame in this process. More total understanding of the deeper meaning behind an illness allows an individual to take responsibility for his/her healthcare on all levels.

The actual phrase "to take responsibility for one's own healthcare" sounds challenging and positive but it can also seem overwhelming and daunting. Individuals will, quite rightly, approach this prospect in varying ways, some with great enthusiasm and some very tentatively. The manner adopted will reflect an individual's attitude of mind, overall state of health and background: each client brings his/her own agenda to a consultation. Ideally, the process can be constructive and worthwhile, bringing an understanding of how we feel when we are well or unwell. Reflexology consultations, along with those of other complementary therapies, create a situation where people can become fully acquainted with themselves.

The ultimate aim is for each person to be aware that, whether they are well or unwell, the whole experience of treatment can be rewarding. If a person has a problem, it is not something alien that needs to be got rid of, but rather, it is an integral part of that individual and, as such, it is something to be understood and accepted. It is not a case of fighting or of being defeated but of accepting while maintaining a strong sense of self and moving forward positively. Also, the state of health at that time is not an isolated incident but part of an ongoing process.

This idea of understanding symptoms, almost of forming a relationship with them, may seem impossible but it can be paralleled to the parent/child relationship that can seem equally impossible at times. Sometimes this can be harmonious and easy and, at other times, it can be challenging and provocative. For any relationship to be worthwhile, it should be dynamic, and constantly changing situations arise that could be potentially confrontational. A child can be controlled and suppressed, providing acceptable and immediate order but also creating a distance between the parent and the child or, alternatively, attention can be given to the child's nature, attempting to understand how the situation arose. This latter approach requires more time and energy and is less conventional. However, ultimately it is more rewarding for all concerned, and certainly the relationship that develops as a result is deeper, stronger and richer and will continue to grow and flourish.

The various elements within precision reflexology treatments, the practitioner's skill and intuitive sense, the client's involvement and the relationship between the client and the therapist, all support the process of understanding and growth.

> *"If you ask for kindness, be kind*
> *If you ask for truth, be true*
> *What you give of yourself, you find*
> *This world is a reflex of you"*

Gandhi

CHAPTER 16

The "unseen": Advanced precision reflexology

As previously described, precision reflexology gives shape and form to one way of working with subtle body energy. There is a stillness to this approach which provides a very welcome relief from the fast pace of modern life. This stillness and the "low-tech" style are therapeutic when taken in the context of the stress and anxiety that many clients experience on a daily basis.

The "unseen" work is a natural development of precision work. It has evolved from the realisation of the value of foot massage as an extremely beneficial procedure. It acknowledges the feet as a powerful medium; the way that they provide a real connection with the true energy of the body in a totally non-invasive way and how they evoke the parasympathetic nervous system to promote a deep sense of relaxation. "Unseen" work embraces both a Western and Eastern view of reflexology. The "hands-on" work is via the feet, using a thorough foot massage sequence with the powerful addition of the subtle energy work of precision reflexology techniques. This is then developed to encompass wider aspects of naturopathic healthcare so that, if they wish, clients can feel involved in, and more aware of, their own health status. In this way, the treatment becomes truly holistic.

In this advanced work, some of the potent "links" of precision work are used. These are combined with a detailed foot massage sequence and then a programme of self-help can be developed as a result of the responses to the treatment. This approach provides a challenging focus for the therapeutic consultation. The links that are used work through the Chakra system of the body so that there is a genuine clarity to the subsequent planning of the healthcare programme, which reasonates with the client in an appropriate and realistic way.

Although "unseen" work can be viewed as a pioneering approach, both the treatment and the self-help advice are based entirely on traditional, well established forms of healthcare. The aim is for the client to feel empowered and to reconnect to old skills, which are economical, realistic and enjoyable. They require an acknowledgement of the value of adopting a slower pace of life from time to time. This can be reflected in the way in which we provide and eat our food, by how we allow ourselves some quiet, reflective time, by how we exercise; in fact by how we look after ourselves physically, emotionally and spiritually. There is a recognition that, often, the old ways are the best!

In common with basic precision reflexology the main principles of "unseen" work are:

- The over-riding aim is to connect to the subtle energy of the body and to help restore balance to the system. This energy is dynamic, energetic and constantly changing. The connection is often deep, working on an unconscious level.
- The treatment aims to be truly holistic in approach and in application.
- There is an awareness that the body has an innate, multi-directional network of communication. This is an intelligent system which exists beyond words and which is not random. This advanced work provides a way to connect to the internal dialogue of a person.
- The subtle energy work requires a light touch and will not respond to heavy physical pressure. "Linking" is used to add power and precision to a treatment and to connect on a subtle level. The two elements of strength and relaxation ideally exist side-by-side in equal measure to create optimum levels of energy, almost as a form of alchemy. This duality, as previously described in Chapter 13, of gentleness and strength, delight and responsibility, can not only co-exist but they actually support each other. This is perfectly summed up by Ralph W. Sockman who said,
  "There is nothing so gentle as true strength and nothing so strong as genuine gentleness."
- Each treatment is unique and appropriate to the client. Treatments proceed at the client's pace, are totally non-invasive and only given when they are welcomed.
- Each "link" is held while the practitioner "listens". Sometimes this intervention prompts a response, a change, but often it is simply the awareness of how energy is functioning that is valuable.
- Sickness in itself is a form of communication. Each person is a location for personal and social harmony, or lack of it. People's health reflects their level of internal and external harmony; of how they relate to themselves and to the world around them. It can indicate whether they exist in a world of struggle and resistance or of creativity and fulfilment.
- The "unseen" approach is that we all have one health which comes with many "ups and downs". Treatment is not about fixing a person or about him/her getting better once and for all. It is about listening, supporting,

and helping people to become involved in their own care, to listen to the "messages" from the body so that they can arrive at a greater understanding and aim to improve their health status.
- The "unseen" approach offers a sense of liberation and freedom to the work of the practitioner. All practitioners can operate within their own field of expertise in order to empower clients.

"Linking" and advanced precision reflexology

As already outlined in Chapter 2, linking relies on the tactile sensitivity of the practitioner. It is intuitive, strong, liberating and creative. It offers a freestyle approach with the minimum of structure. To summarise, the main principles specifically for linking are:
- It is important to maintain a light, energetic touch. Soft fingers, hands, wrists, elbows and shoulders allow a connection with the subtle energy of the body.
- Once a connection has been achieved, the practitioner can then observe and "listen". There is no measurement, no analysis – just intuition and attention. It can feel like a meditation for the practitioner with connections being made on all levels.
- In advanced precision work, the wider aspects of complementary health and the self-help programme that can be discussed with clients are based on the observations of the "linking" procedures.
- The treatment develops at the client's pace and does not involve the will of the practitioner. As with all energy work, it is vital to have clear boundaries about the actual process. Precision reflexology intervention uses a definite tactile contact but it is also clear that there is no energy exchange between the client and the therapist. There is genuine attention but also it is very clear where one person begins and the other ends.

The links used in advanced precision reflexology:

These are based on the reflex points associated with the Chakra system, there are:
1. Base Chakra – ovary to uterus link (see Chapter 10)
2. Sacral Chakra – adrenal to groin link (see Chapter 9)
3. Solar plexus Chakra – solar plexus to itself link (see Chapter 6).
4. Heart Chakra – thymus to itself link (see Chapter 11)
5. Throat Chakra – thyroid to itself link (see Chapter 3)

6. Brow Chakra – Pituitary to adrenal link (see Chapter 3)
7. Crown chakra – Pineal to base of spine link (see Chapter 3)
    The wonder of precision work is that the links provide the tactile contact with the subtle energy of the body.

Procedure

The actual procedure of the "unseen" treatment is, within a massage sequence, to work through these seven links, starting at the Base Chakra on the right foot, up through to the Crown Chakra. Then, on the left foot, starting at the Crown Chakra and working down to the Base. This is a familiar Chakra clearing, grounding and balancing technique. Throughout the treatment the links are interspersed with a full range of massage strokes.

The massage strokes

Foot massage recognises the value of touch as a therapeutic intervention in itself. The sense of touch is the most heightened sense when we are born. Touch is so central to our well-being that without it we can become depressed, anxious and irritable. Massage satisfies our need for touch in a reassuring, supportive way within comfortable limits. Massage has been used throughout history by many cultures both as a form of prevention and of treatment of illness. It is an intuitive, powerful form of communication which does not need words.

There are, of course, many and varied massage strokes and many of these can be used in "unseen" work. This allows practitioners to be creative and to develop their own procedure. As with all massage sequences it is important to maintain a sense of fluidity and flow to the treatment. Also the therapeutic benefits are enhanced by including a variety of strokes to include effleurage, petrissage, percussion and mobilisation techniques. In addition, by completing a thorough treatment with a full range of strokes, it can be seen that in reflexology terms, the reflexes associated with the whole body have been worked.

Definitions of massage strokes

Effleurage – these long, smoothing strokes are often used by way of a gentle introduction to massage. They follow on from each other, helping to increase their beneficial effects and they also blend sequences together, allowing them to feel soothing and relaxing.

Percussion – these movements improve muscle tone and are invigorating and warming. They loosen tight structures with a sense of vibration. These stimulating strokes are often used at the end of a treatment to assist the transition back into everyday awareness.

Mobilisation – these are passive exercises which can be used to free tension from structures.

Petrissage – these detailed, superficial strokes are used sensitively to ease out tension and to improve circulation.

Examples of strokes for foot massages

Effluerage
Double-handed effleurage from toes to ankle
Horizontal strokes with both thumbs over whole of plantar surface
Rake over the dorsal surface with soft fingers from ankle to toes
Double handed effleurage of fingers to work from the toes to the ankle

Percussion
Web of hand working the Achilles area
"Train" – circular movements with palm of hands work down both sides of feet from toes to heel
"Bounces" – with soft palms, bounce the sides of the foot from one hand to the other
Gentle slaps over plantar surface

Petrissage
Edge of knuckles work around the reflex for the pelvic area
Knuckles of fist work down plantar surface from toes to heel
Circular thumb pressures work over reflexes for spinal muscles
On dorsal surface, thumb pressures work down from ankle to toes – and then effleurage back to ankle
"Breaking bread" – hold foot in both hands with thumbs on plantar and fingers on dorsal. Alternately apply pressure from the thumbs and then from the fingers to create an arch shape
"Corkscrew" – use knuckle of forefinger to work over the area at the base of the toes on plantar surface

Mobilisation
Flex and stretch movements of the ankle joint
Rotation of the ankle joint
Hold heel and gently twist top third of foot from side to side
Rotate and stretch each toe in turn
Throughout the sequence, general effleurage can be interspersed with other strokes

The Chakras

As already discussed in Chapter 3, the Chakras can represent one way to define the subtle energy of the body. Individually the Chakras offer a way to describe different aspects of one united energy. Collectively they are a "bridge" between the physical, emotional, mental and spiritual aspects of ourselves. The movement of that energy is what makes us all unique. The Chakras need not be remote or alien; they are simply a form of language, they are representations of our holistic nature.

Interestingly, the presence of neuropeptides in the body, as described in Chapter 3, could be a Western model for this concept. We know that the nervous, endocrine and immune systems all interact with each other. The emotions and bodily sensations are intertwined, in a two-way network where each can alter the other. This integration is called the psychoimmunoendocrine network. The immune system communicates with the endocrine and nervous systems using the neuropeptides; like other body chemicals these help to regulate various body processes. The significance of neuropeptides is that they are found in various locations in the body and they all have receptors in the brain. The excitement is that this offers a scientific explanation for the holistic approach that believes the physical body can retain emotions and is affected by them. It is impossible to separate the body, the mind and the spirit as they all affect each other constantly; they are always communicating. Likewise neuropeptides and their receptors communicate between the brain, the glands, the nerves and the immune system.

There is a great resonance with the Chakras and the endocrine system; they are not the same but the characteristics of each have many similarities. Energy moves between the Chakras, which are constantly changing, adapting and responding to each other in the same way that hormone levels throughout the endocrine system respond to each other. The nature of the "unseen" treatment itself is fluid, flexible and intuitive.

The essence of advanced precision reflexology focuses on the subtle energy of the body in general and on the identity of each Chakra in particular. It is called the "unseen" because it aims to connect to the unseen nature within. Therefore it is central to this approach to look at the nature of each Chakra.

Base Chakra – Muladhara

The location of this is thought to be at the base of the spine in the perineum. The characteristics include security, survival instincts, creativity, constructive thought, vitality and the ability to live in the present moment. Its physical counterpart is the gonads. To relate this to the therapeutic consultation, if a client is low in spirit and sees day-to-day life as a chore, then it would be fair to assume that there would be an imbalance on this chakra and the "link" that could detect this would be the ovary to uterus for women or testicle to prostate for men. There may not be a physical problem with that area but any imbalance could reflect the emotions of that area; this applies to all the "unseen" links. The healing process involves holding the "link" and aiming to restore a sense of balance, on all levels. The colour that is associated with this Chakra is red.

Sacrum Chakra – Svadisthana

This is associated with the sacrum and the physical counterpart within the endocrine system is the adrenal glands. The nature of this is courage, the fight/flight syndrome and also social interaction. The "link" that can have a positive effect therapeutically is the adrenal to groin one. Again, to relate this to the forum of the consultation, if a client is often fearful of life situations or expresses regret as a result of being afraid to take opportunities, an imbalance with this link will be felt. The colour for this Chakra is orange.

Note that there is a reciprocal energy between the first and second chakra so sometimes the characteristics overlap between the two. One explanation for this is that in comparison to the dense structure of the sacrum, the base of the spine is more delicate to allow our energy to be grounded to the earth.

Solar Plexus Chakra – Manipura

This is thought to be situated in the solar plexus area of the body and the endocrine gland associated with it is the pancreas. Its identity is one of self-esteem, confidence and the ability to control situations. The "link" for this is the solar plexus to itself. Clients who lack confidence will often present with an imbalance in the vibrations felt on this link. The rounded shoulder posture of someone who is feeling a lack of confidence shows how, instinctively, we try to protect the vulnerable area. Also it is common to have a craving for sweet food when confidence is low; perhaps this is this Chakra, and its partner gland, asking for some attention? The associated colour is yellow.

Heart Chakra – Anahata

This is associated with the heart and its gland is the thymus. This gives us our sense of belonging, identity with self, security, sense of compassion and our ability to form relationships. The "link" is the thymus to itself. If a client has a problem with a relationship or if they are suffering from any form of grief or loss surrounding a relationship, then an imbalance on this link will be felt. An example of the gland/Chakra partnership is demonstrated when people who are grieving often become ill as the thymus struggles with its role in the immune system. The colour for this Chakra is green.

Throat Chakra – Vishuddi

This is thought to be situated in the throat area of the body. Its associated gland is the thyroid. It offers social order, the ability to express oneself and communication skills in general. The "link" is the thyroid to itself. Any imbalances that are felt may indicate a lack of communication with the outside world or within the individual – for instance, if a client finds it difficult to make connections between the physical, emotional and spiritual parts of him/herself. The colour for this one is blue.

Brow Chakra – Ajna

This is thought to be situated in the centre of the forehead and is sometimes called the "Third Eye". It is partnered with the pituitary gland. It provides inventive thought, our awareness of the future and our sense of intuition. The "link" for this is the pituitary to adrenal. This link perfectly demonstrates the connection between the physical body and subtle energy. In Chapter 3, it was explained that this link can assist with problems with the menopause by encouraging the pituitary to reduce the over-activity of the adrenal glands. On a subtle level, the increased activity of the sacrum Chakra reflects the fear that is often present at this time of life. This can be offset by stimulating the brow Chakra and encouraging the woman to be more aware of her wisdom and intuitive skills. In common with some other cultures of the world, it focuses on the positive aspects of the menopause rather than the negative which is often the conventional view in the West. This Chakra's colour is indigo.

Crown Chakra – Sahasrara

This is associated with the crown of the head and its gland is the pineal. It gives us our artistic expression, imagery skills and our overall sense of spirituality. It is activated during meditation. Its gland is the pineal. The "link" is the pineal to the base of the spine. The link provides a sense of balance, aiming to ground someone who had "their head in the clouds" or to lift someone's spirits who was "down in the dumps". The associated colour is violet.

The Chakras, as centres of energy, can be seen to correspond to the curves of the spine; they exist in relation to our structure (see *Figure 16.1*). The "unseen" work gives a practical aspect to something that is often perceived as being very impractical. It provides a structure and form to intuitive, energetic therapy work. It offers a tactile contact, via "linking", with the subtle body.

Just to reiterate, consistent tenderness on the links associated with the glands and the Chakras, which does not seem to have any physical basis could be explained in terms of the subtle body. For example, a painful,

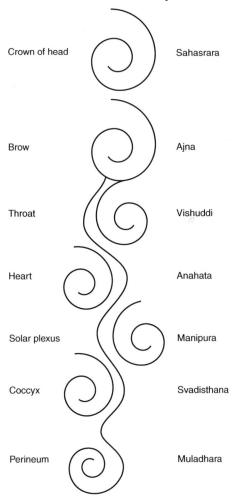

Crown of head — Sahasrara

Brow — Ajna

Throat — Vishuddi

Heart — Anahata

Solar plexus — Manipura

Coccyx — Svadisthana

Perineum — Muladhara

Figure 16.1: Chakras in relation to the spine.

tender reaction or an imbalance felt by the practitioner on the thyroid link, may indicate that the person has a difficulty with some aspect of communication. The response relates to the emotionality of the organ rather than to its physicality.

The ethos of the treatment is simply one of acceptance, there need be no analysis, just observation.

"Unseen" foot chart

These are not charts as such but rather pictures of the feet which show reflex points that offer connections to the Chakra system. There are no anatomical reflex points at all. The position of the points shown in *Figure 16.2* is based on the energetic responses that relate to each Chakra. Each Chakra is present on both feet but, for clarity in the diagram, they are shown just once spread over both feet.

As previously explained, the tactile contact with this way of working is based around a thorough foot massage sequence which is interspersed with the links that are associated with each Chakra. These Chakra points are worked from the base up to the crown on the right foot and then from the crown down to the base on the left foot.

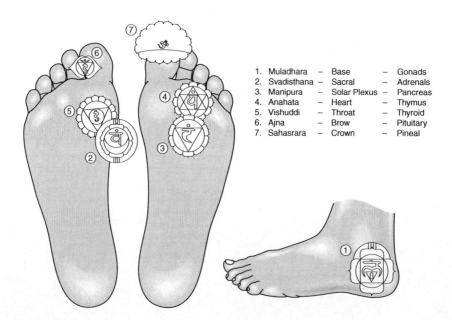

1.	Muladhara	–	Base	–	Gonads
2.	Svadisthana	–	Sacral	–	Adrenals
3.	Manipura	–	Solar Plexus	–	Pancreas
4.	Anahata	–	Heart	–	Thymus
5.	Vishuddi	–	Throat	–	Thyroid
6.	Ajna	–	Brow	–	Pituitary
7.	Sahasrara	–	Crown	–	Pineal

Figure 16.2: The "unseen" chart.

Wider aspects of "unseen" work – the self-help programmes

One of the distinguishing features of complementary healthcare is that clients are encouraged to have a greater sense of awareness and involvement in their own healthcare. The therapeutic consultation provides an ideal forum for the therapist to discuss with clients how they can adopt appropriate methods of self-care in their everyday lives. Obviously the advice given needs to be based on professional expertise and it also needs to be realistic and enjoyable so that it can be sustained and become part of a daily routine.

Obviously, there is a beneficial intervention provided by the hands-on treatment itself: the 'linking' technique aims to restore balance to each Chakra point, addressing the elements that are relevant to each recipient of the treatment. The "unseen" work, in common with all precision reflexology, connects to the true, essential energy of each person. Practitioners can then use their own skill and expertise to plan, with the client, a programme of care that will resonate on a deep, authentic level. The client can then continue the intent of the treatment in their own time. The excitement of "unseen" work is that any imbalances have been related to individual chakras, to specific aspects of the subtle body, and any self-help programme will also resonate in the same way. Therapists use their own knowledge of a modality, and the nature of each Chakra, to advise clients on self-help procedures that aim to re-dress any imbalances that were felt during the treatment. Experienced practitioners also work with their knowledge of clients so that any advice will be compatible with their lifestyle, ability, overall state of health and personal preferences. Obviously practitioners can only work within their own field of expertise and skill so that they are fully aware of any possible contraindications. The focus is to identify the specific elements of each modality that will resonate with the vibrations of the relevant Chakra.

Some of the modalities that have been used in "unseen" work include nutrition, breathing techniques, yoga-based exercises, affirmations, aromatherapy, colour therapy and crystal therapy.

The following table illustrate two examples, aromatherapy and the use of affirmations:

Chakra	Identity	Aromatherapy oil	Affirmation theme
Base	Vitality	Sandalwood	Joy of life
Sacrum	Courage	Neroli	Bravery
Solar plexus	Confidence	Lemongrass	Self-esteem
Heart	Relationships	Rose	Love/belonging
Throat	Communication	Lavender	Self-expression
Brow	Intuition	Chamomile	Trust of intuition
Crown	Spirituality	Frankincense	Sense of spirit

Using these two examples, if an imbalance had been felt on the throat Chakra, the practitioner could have encouraged the client to make, in their own words, a positive statement about communication. The client can then practice this whenever he/she feels the need to.

Or, if the therapist is also an aromatherapist, the client would have been advised on the home use of lavender oil.

The creativity of this approach is that therapists can devise their own treatment plans. The therapist also can decide which approach is most appropriate for each client. The dialogue surrounding these self-help programmes will vary from one client to another, depending on how comfortable each client is with the concept of subtle energy. The consultation remains the central reference point so that, at subsequent treatments, clients can report back on their progress and any necessary adaptations can be made.

Thus advanced precision reflexology, the "unseen" work, asks for an open-minded approach and an open-hearted one too. It is intuitive, accepting and supportive in manner. It has the ability to connect to the heart and soul of the client – and also to the practitioner.

References

Montague A (1986) *Touching*. Harper and Row, USA: 163

Pert CB (1998) *Molecules of Emotion*. Simon and Schuster, New York: 307

Smith FF (1998) *Inner Bridges*. Humanics Ltd, USA: 54

Recommended reading

Colburn T, Myers JP, Dumanoski D (1996) *Stolen Future*. Little Brown and Company, USA

Cormack M, Mitchell A (1998) *The Therapeutic Relationship in Complementary Health Care*. Churchill Livingstone, Edinburgh

Frawley D, Lad V (2004) *The Yoga of Herbs*. Lotus Light Publications, USA

Holford P (1997) *The Optimum Nutrition Bible*. Piatkus, London

Issel C (1990) *Reflexology, Art, Science and History*. New Frontier, Sacramento, California

Lawrence F (2008) *Eat Your Heart Out*. Penguin books, London

Mackereth and Tiran (2010) *Clinical Reflexology*. Churchill Livingstone, Edinburgh

Mitchell S (1998) *Naturopathy*. Element Books, Shaftesbury

Montagu A (1986) *Touching*. Harper and Row, USA

Pert CB (1998) *Molecules of Emotion*. Simon and Schuster, USA

Sivananda Yoga Centre (Lidell, Rabinovitch and Rabinovitch) (1993) The Book of Yoga. Ebury Press, London

Smith FF (1998) *Inner Bridges*. Humanics Ltd, USA

Uhl M (1996) *Chakra Energy Massage*. Lotus Light Publications, USA

Useful addresses

Federation of Precision Reflexology

Email – jan@precisionreflexology.com

Association of Reflexologists

5 Fore Street

Taunton

Somerset TA1 1HX

Email – info@aor.org.uk

Index

J

jaw 28

L

leg reflexes on the feet 30
life-style changes 79
linking 13, 14–15, 65, 82 83
  technique 28
lumbar 5/hip link 46
lumbar 5/hip/sciatic loop 57–60

M

Manipura 87
massage 84
  examples of strokes 85
menopause 53
menstruation 33–35
mobilisation 85
movement 33
Muladhara 86

N

naturopathic healthcare 81
neck 28

O

ovary to uterus link 53, 55
ovary to uterus to pituitary link 55

P

parathyroid 19–20
percussion 85
  massage 65
petrissage 85
phlebitis 20
pineal 11–16, 20
pituitary 12–14
precision reflexology 23
  advanced 83
  chart 68
  procedure 72
  techniques 62

R

radiotherapy 72
reflexology
  contraindications 72
relaxation 74, 81

S

sacrum Chakra 87
Sahasrara 88
self-help 61, 73, 91
senses 34
sensory organs
  reflexes for 47
shoulder link 27
sinusitis 27
skeleton system 41
  links 43
solar plexus 87
spinal reflexes 43
Stkira 69, 75
stress 75
Svadisthana 87

T

Tai Chi 74
Third Eye 88
throat Chakra 88
thymus 19, 57
thyroid 20, 72
thyroxin 62
tinnitus 61

U

"unseen"
  foot chart 90
  work 82

V

Vishuddi 88

Y

Yoga 74